HORIZONS IN CANCER RESEARCH

HORIZONS IN CANCER RESEARCH

VOLUME 73

HORIZONS IN CANCER RESEARCH

Additional books and e-books in this series can be found on Nova's website under the Series tab.

HORIZONS IN CANCER RESEARCH

HORIZONS IN CANCER RESEARCH

VOLUME 73

HIROTO S. WATANABE
EDITOR

nova
Medicine & Health

Library of Congress Cataloging-in-Publication Data

ISBN: 978-1-53616-273-8
ISSN: 2159-1326

Published by Nova Science Publishers, Inc. † New York

CONTENTS

PREFACE

In Horizons in Cancer Research. Volume 73, after the identification of some small subgroups with a strong biological-molecular identity, the current evidence regarding the prognostic factors of patients with non-eradicable metastatic disease are examined. The goal is to discuss disease subgroups, which may sometimes provide conditions for decisions that are less compliant with current clinical practice and help define new stratification criteria for patients enrolled in prospective studies.

Following this, the authors summarize the current knowledge on breast cancer with an introduction on the traditional markers used in the diagnosis of this disease, followed by an account of the emerging markers.

Next, the underlying mechanisms of DNA replication, damage and repair are discussed. Further, RAD51 is proposed as a potential means of managing chemoresistant cancers. Certain drugs and strategies can sensitize chemotherapy via impacting on RAD51, which can be developed as chemotherapy modulators.

The authors also discuss multiple myeloma, an incurable malignant tumor of plasma cells of the bone marrow, which is the most common primary neoplasm arising in bone. It causes approximately 1% of cancer-related deaths and is the 2nd most common hematological malignancy in the western world.

Later, this collection discusses the prevalence and types of infectious complications that patients with multiple myeloma face, as well as present and emerging therapeutic approaches.

The concluding study indicates proteins that have a promising future as new anticancer drugs, in conjunction with the in vitro and/or in vivo effects of these bioactive proteins derived from plants.

Chapter 1 - The high lethality rate of pancreatic adenocarcinoma (PDAC) leads more than 90% of patients inevitably to experience a non-eradicable metastatic disease (mPDAC). Not much has changed between 1997 and 2017 regarding the course of mPDAC, whose optimal median expected overall survival passed from 4.4 to 11.8 months; in addition, however, some studies hypothesize that the median survival is much lower in clinical practice, also due to an excess of early deaths. Furthermore, mPDAC is probably the clinical setting in medical oncology in which the highest rate of failures for targeted drugs and immunotherapy has been recorded, so much so that the drugs approved to date are almost exclusively cytotoxic agents.

In conjunction with the frustrating efforts to improve therapeutic armament, even in the most recent studies, a consistent progress in the variables related to survival has not been done, and the prognostic factors accepted by all the authors remain the performance status and the extent of disease, while other clinical factors are not widely recognized. The contradictory evidence on the prognostic role is also common for most molecular biological variables, for which is added the great difficulty of obtaining sufficient samples for the diagnosis, the pathological and molecular determinations. In this context, the recent molecular classification of PDAC by the ICGC has changed little the understanding and clinical management of the metastatic disease.

After the identification of some small subgroups with a strong biological-molecular identity (MMR-deficient, BRCA-mutated, etc.), the current evidences about the prognostic factors of patients with mPDAC are examined, with the purpose of discussing, and possibly characterize disease subgroups, which may sometimes provide the conditions for decisions that are less “compliant” with current clinical practice and help define new stratification criteria for patients enrolled in prospective studies.

Chapter 2 - Worldwide statistics suggest that breast cancer is the commonest cancer among women, accounting for nearly 25% of the total cancer cases. Though the survival rate is higher in the developed countries, it is poorer in the developing countries. Risk factors include advanced age, lack of childbearing and breastfeeding, Western dietary patterns and obesity, hormonal factors and genetic factors. Genetic factors include BRCA1 and BRCA2 gene mutations, and mutations/alterations in p53, PTEN, STK11, CHEK2, ATM, BRIK1 and PALB2 genes, and changes in DNA-repair genes like MSH2 and MLH1.

The advent of protein and DNA arrays and metabolomics platforms have led to accumulation of an immense amount of data, thereby providing crucial knowledge on the genetic signature of various types of breast cancer, and facilitating molecular diagnosis and therapy. Besides this, gene expression profiling and real-time PCR arrays are also used to explore cancer signaling pathways. Further, epigenetic markers have been discovered which are characteristic of certain breast cancer sub-types. . The challenge currently is to validate the utility of these markers. In future, Microarray-based and proteomic studies are expected to explore utilities and unearth new markers.

This chapter summarizes the current knowledge on the subject with an introduction on the “traditional” markers used in the diagnosis of breast cancer, followed by an account of the emerging markers

Chapter 3 - Cancer commonly has a high level of DNA replication, damage and repair. RAD51 plays an important role in homologous recombination, a pathway of DNA repair. Recent data have manifested that RAD51 is involved in platinum resistance in ovarian cancer. Platinum agents induce DNA breaks; therefore, DNA repair may lead to cell survival, and eventually results in treatment failure. Here underlying mechanisms are discussed in brief. Further, RAD51 is a potential target to manage chemoresistant cancers. Certain drugs and strategies can sensitize chemotherapy via impacting on RAD51, which can be developed as chemotherapy modulators.

Chapter 4 - Multiple myeloma (MM) is an incurable malignant tumor of plasma cells of the bone marrow and is the most common primary neoplasm arising in bone. It causes approximately 1% of cancer-related deaths and is the 2nd commonest hematological malignancy in the western world. The median age at diagnosis is 69 years and it is an infrequent diagnosis before the age of 40 years.

Although the etiology of MM is not well-understood, it is thought to arise as a result of multiple genetic mutations of plasma cells and the immunoglobulins they produce. Some studies also suggest an association with occupational and environmental risk factors. Abnormalities of chromosome 13 are also detected in approximately 50% patients with MM.

Pathological fractures occur in approximately 40% patients. Bone disease also causes bone pain, spinal cord compression, diffuse osteoporosis and hypercalcemia, compromising mortality, morbidity and quality of life. Anemia, renal dysfunction and hypercalcemia are common metabolic complications and can range from mild to life-threatening. Immunosuppression, due to the disease itself and its treatment, can lead to frequent infections. Diagnosis depends on detection of M-proteins in plasma or urine, bone marrow biopsy, and end organ or bone damage.

Although MM remains incurable, improvements in treatment have had favorable impact on survival rates. Typical treatment combines alkylating chemotherapy drugs (Melaphan, Doxorubicin or Cyclophosphamide), a steroid (Dexamethazone or Prednisolone) and an immunomodulatory agent (Thalidomide, Lenalidomide or Bortezomib), depending on age and co-morbidities of the patients. Bisphosphonates are recommended for use in all symptomatic patients, of which Zoledronate and Pamidronate have proven efficacy. Radiotherapy is used to control pain and palliative treatment of focal lesions of disseminated disease.

Surgery has a supportive effect on long-term survival rates and quality of life in myeloma patients. Surgery is considered palliative in the majority of cases and surgical risks must be weighed against life expectancy and quality of life to justify surgical intervention. Stem cell transplantation combined with chemotherapy can be considered the standard of care in patients up to 65 years. Prognosis is highly variable, with overall estimated 35% survival at 5-years and 17% at 10-years with newer treatments.

Chapter 5 - Multiple myeloma, a hematological malignancy characterized by the proliferation of malignant plasma cells within the bone marrow, is associated with reduced immunity. Multiple myeloma related immunodeficiency involves B-cell dysfunction and abnormalities of T-cells, dendritic cells, and NK-cells. The literature shows that patients with multiple myeloma display a low immune response to infections and vaccines, have a higher risk of infection, and most importantly, note that infectious diseases are the leading cause of death in these patients. Recent studies have reported an evolving range of infections in multiple myeloma, likely due to new therapies including stem cell therapies, novel agents, and monoclonal antibodies. This book chapter will briefly review the prevalence and types of infectious complications that patients with multiple myeloma face as well as present and emerging therapeutic approaches.

Chapter 6 - Plants are rich sources of compounds with varied structures and potent biological effects against diseases, including cancer. Many studies have been performed to investigate plant-derived compounds with the ability to impair tumor formation or control cancer progression such as lectins (carbohydrate-binding proteins). This review discusses the *in vitro* and/or *in vivo* effects of these bioactive proteins from plants against cancer cells or models. Lectins interfere with cell growth and survival by binding to specific membrane receptors or internalization via endocytosis. In both cases, they can block the pathways involved in cell growth and survival (e.g., PI3K/Akt/mTOR, ERK, and NF-κB signaling), induce oxidative stress, trigger apoptosis through the induction of an imbalance of pro-apoptotic and anti-apoptotic proteins and/or the activation of death receptors, induce autophagy-related gene expression, and cause necrosis. Although some lectins have been studied in clinical trials, there are many others that deserve attention. The current study indicates such proteins that have a promising future as new anticancer drugs.

In: Horizons in Cancer Research. Volume 73 ISBN: 978-1-53616-273-8
Editor: Hiroto S. Watanabe

Chapter 1

CURRENT VIEWS ON PROGNOSTIC FACTORS OF PATIENTS WITH METASTATIC PANCREATIC ADENOCARCINOMA

Giuseppe A. Colloca**, MD, Antonella Venturino, MD and Domenico Guarneri, MD
Oncologia Medica Imperiese (OMI), Imperia, Italy

ABSTRACT

The high lethality rate of pancreatic adenocarcinoma (PDAC) leads more than 90% of patients inevitably to experience a non-eradicable metastatic disease (mPDAC). Not much has changed between 1997 and 2017 regarding the course of mPDAC, whose optimal median expected overall survival passed from 4.4 to 11.8 months; in addition, however, some studies hypothesize that the median survival is much lower in clinical practice, also due to an excess of early deaths. Furthermore, mPDAC is probably the clinical setting in medical oncology in which the highest rate of failures for targeted drugs and immunotherapy has been recorded, so

* Corresponding Author's E-mail: g.colloca@katamail.com.

much so that the drugs approved to date are almost exclusively cytotoxic agents.

In conjunction with the frustrating efforts to improve therapeutic armament, even in the most recent studies, a consistent progress in the variables related to survival has not been done, and the prognostic factors accepted by all the authors remain the performance status and the extent of disease, while other clinical factors are not widely recognized. The contradictory evidence on the prognostic role is also common for most molecular biological variables, for which is added the great difficulty of obtaining sufficient samples for the diagnosis, the pathological and molecular determinations. In this context, the recent molecular classification of PDAC by the ICGC has changed little the understanding and clinical management of the metastatic disease.

After the identification of some small subgroups with a strong biological-molecular identity (MMR-deficient, BRCA-mutated, etc.), the current evidences about the prognostic factors of patients with mPDAC are examined, with the purpose of discussing, and possibly characterize disease subgroups, which may sometimes provide the conditions for decisions that are less "compliant" with current clinical practice and help define new stratification criteria for patients enrolled in prospective studies.

INTRODUCTION

Pancreatic cancer is the seventh leading cause of global cancer deaths worldwide (Rawla 2019). From the year 2017 deaths from pancreatic cancer (PDAC) are more than deaths from breast cancer in European Union (91500 vs. 91000) (Ferlay 2017), and a similar trend has been registered in United States (41780 vs. 40890) (Siegel 2016). In the United States in 2019 about 56770 new cases of pancreatic cancer have been estimated, accounting the 3.2% of all new cancer cases; estimated deaths in 2019 are 45750, equal to 7.5% of all cancer deaths, and, from 2009 to 2015 9.3% is the percent surviving 5 years (Cancer Stat Facts 2019). Despite the survival improvements reported for all stages of PDAC, the mortality rate remains very close to that of incidence. This picture depends on the fact that about 80-85% of patients with PDAC are diagnosed with metastatic or unresectable disease (Li 2004), and only 20% have a potentially curable disease. But even for patients diagnosed with localized PDAC, 5-year survival is 25-30% (Katz 2009), although further improvement is possible in the near future thanks to new regimens of adjuvant chemotherapy (Conroy 2018). However, even among patients undergoing radical surgery, PDAC mortality exceeds that for other causes up to 8.75 years after diagnosis (Swords 2018).

These data make us understand that the development of early metastases is a common phenomenon for PDAC, which occurs in over 80% of cases at diagnosis as an unresectable tumor. Along this paper we will discuss about locally advanced or metastatic pancreatic cancer (mPDAC) due to this is the definition commonly used in clinical trials, even though the expected median overall survival (OS) of mPDAC fluctuates between 6-11 months in the presence of metastasis (Conroy 2011) up to 12-16 months of the unresectable locally-advanced disease (Hammel 2016).

PROGNOSTIC FACTORS OF MPDAC

In this chapter, we will focus on the prognosis and analysis of prognostic factors (PFs) related to patients with mPDAC, for which to date only cytotoxic drugs are approved, and for which from 1990 to 2011 the standard of care was mono-chemotherapy. The only non-cytotoxic drug to demonstrate a benefit in addition to gemcitabine was erlotinib: the combination was studied in 569 patients with mPDAC and was associated with a small increase of median OS from 5.91 to 6.24 months (Moore 2007). Given the poor prognosis and the very slow improvement of medical therapies, the development of new PFs of mPDAC has been slow too.

A prognostic factor is any variable, usually related to the tumor or to the patient, that is able to modify the outcome independently of the other variables. The clinical importance of PFs lies in the fact that they help patients avoid unnecessary toxicity and complications from aggressive treatments, while they are essential for the progress of clinical research because they allow stratification of the sample in trials. Unlike the predictive factor, which predicts the efficacy of a treatment in a patient population, PF independently predicts survival, regardless of treatments, but also of other variables. One of the critical issues in clinical oncology is the standardization of prognostic variables, and mPDAC is no exception: in fact, these variables vary greatly between prospective phase-3 studies, and many PFs are questionable since they have been identified in uncontrolled studies, with limited case numbers and inadequate statistical power. Since the phase-3 prospective randomized trials (RCTs) remain the most objective method for evaluating the efficacy of antineoplastic treatments, they are also the most important and reliable source of information on PFs. Indeed, in RCTs, the evaluation of all variables that influence survival, and are independent of the treatment arm, is essential to support the conclusions of the study. However, these analyses are not always obvious and with the same results over time, so the change in PDAC epidemiology, treatments or diagnostic procedures can affect the weight of the various PFs.

Also in mPDAC many variables have been evaluated to predict prognosis, and over time have been tested in RCTs in addition to the treatment arm, but, despite the relative homogeneity of the types of studies and treatments that have occurred along 20 years, PFs on which to design future clinical studies have not been uniquely defined. Taking into account this unanswered need to have reliable variables on which to design studies of mPDAC, a recent consensus statement on mandatory measurements in pancreatic cancer trials (COMM-PACT) has come to important conclusions. The consensus has begun its review process with an analysis of the most commonly reported PFs in 39 RCTs from 2000 to 2016. These variables were then subjected to expert evaluation using a modified Delphi panel of two rounds involving 23 leading medical oncologists in the field of PDAC. The authors concluded that only 12 PFs could be considered as mandatory (age, albumin, bilirubin, CA 19-9, C-reactive protein (CRP), disease status, lactate dehydrogenase (LDH), liver metastasis, neutrophil-to-lymphocyte ratio, number of metastatic sites, pain at baseline, performance status) for future RCTs, while other 8 variables were only recommended (alkaline phosphatase, sex, primary tumor location, pulmonary metastasis, previous deep venous thrombosis or embolus, quality of life-global, quality of life-physical functioning, synchronous or metachronous metastases) (ter Veer 2018).

Table 1. Results of the variables reporting a prognostic role after multivariate analysis in the 13 selected trials

Variable	No. trials	Confirming trials	Not confirming trials
Performance status	13	8	5
Stage III vs. IV	8	7	1
Age	6	1	5
Sex	5	1	4
Albumin	4	2	2
Pain	3	3	0
Liver metastases	3	3	0
Baseline CA 19-9	3	1	2
Tumor site (head vs. body-tail)	2	1	1
Baseline CEA	1	1	0
Weight loss	1	1	0
Timing of metastases	1	1	0
Local diffusion (T4)	1	1	0
Baseline bilirubin	1	1	0
Baseline ALP	1	1	0
Baseline AST	1	1	0

Legend. ALP, alkaline phosphatase. AST, aspartate transaminase. CA 19-9, carbohydrate antigen 19-9. CEA, carcinoembryonic antigen.

Since meta-analyses and RCTs represent the highest level of scientific evidence, in this chapter we have based the analysis of PFs on the latter ones. Therefore, a systematic review of all the RCTs that studied first-line medical therapies in patients with mPDAC allowed us to select 37 studies, published from 1997 to 2017. In 18/37 a PF analysis was performed, but only 13 studies report the results of a multivariate analysis, that took into account all the variables and defined which of them could be considered independent PF (Ducreux 2002; Maisey 2002; Moore 2003; Van Cutsem 2004; Oettle 2005; Louvet 2005; Moore 2007; Herrmann 2007; Poplin 2009; Colucci 2010; Kindler 2011; Conroy 2011; Von Hoff 2013). With all the limitations related to the analysis of the PFs, which were arbitrarily included in the evaluations of the single studies, this review led to the results summarized in Table 1. In it are listed all the PFs that have shown an independent role in at least one study, and the number of studies that have confirmed (confirming trials) or not (not confirming trials) their relationship with OS after multivariate analysis.

Performance Status

Performance status (PS) represents a global assessment by the physician of the patient's functional level, it has been extensively evaluated in oncology outpatient settings both to assess eligibility for clinical studies and to determine the level of fitness towards antineoplastic treatments, as well as to assess the response to treatments. The PS scales according to Karnofsky (Karnofsky 1949) or to Eastern Cooperative Oncology Group (ECOG) (Oken 1982) have been developed mainly to evaluate the ability of cancer patients to tolerate cytotoxic chemotherapy. In particular, in the PDAC, regardless of the stage the PS appears to be the most important PF ever (Tas 2013).

Of the 13 RCTs of patients with mPDAC, which reported a multivariate analysis of the PFs, all included the PS and 8 confirmed the independent prognostic role for PS (Maisey 2002; Van Cutsem 2004; Oettle 2005; Louvet 2005; Herrmann 2007; Colucci 2010; Kindler 2011; Von Hoff 2013). This confirmation has been reported, even though this parameter was evaluated with different scales within the 8 studies (Karnofsky in 3, ECOG in 5).

As with most solid tumors, patients with poor PS usually do not benefit from a combination or intensified chemotherapy regimens and have a poorer prognosis. This last effect is independent of age, stage (Tas 2013), line of medical therapy (Lim 2011; Tanaka 2008), activation of the systemic inflammatory response (Kadokura 2016). A meta-analysis of 14 studies found that there is often a significant positive correlation between PS and patient-reported outcomes (PROs), although this occurred only in 14/18 studies (Atkinson 2015). For this reason, the correlation studies between PS and PROs are interesting, and among the most studied PROs, those related to the quality of life are frequently investigated, both as a PF and as an endpoint of clinical studies of mPDAC (Chiorean 2018). Though the relationship between PS and OS during cytotoxic chemotherapy is strong, it could not be confirmed after other therapies, as it has been reported for targeted therapies in other tumors (Inoue 2009), suggesting that treatment could modify PS and, consequently, reduce or eliminate its prognostic value (Langer 2009). Ultimately, the variable appears susceptible to improvements: in addition to better understanding the differences between PS reported by the doctor with respect to that reported by the patient, increasing attention is paid to distinguishing worsening of the PS linked to the tumor compared to that resulting from other variables (age, comorbidities, polypharmacy, systemic inflammation response, etc.) (Laird 2016), although this distinction sometimes appears almost impossible.

Metastatic vs. Locally Advanced Disease

Of the 13 selected RCTs, 8 included the extent of the disease among the variables subjected to multivariate analysis, and 7 confirmed the significant relationship between mPDAC extension and prognosis (Ducreux 2002; Moore 2003; Van Cutsem 2004; Louvet 2005; Herrmann 2007; Colucci 2010; Kindler 2011), and even a study found that the extent of the primary tumor (category T4 by TNM staging system) was associated with the prognosis independently (Louvet 2005).

More recent studies are increasingly focusing on locally advanced disease (Hammel 2016) or metastatic disease (Conroy 2011). In fact, although locally-advanced and metastatic PDAC appear associated in a single sample in many studies, the locally-advanced disease could benefit from further treatments as well as the systemic one, which could have consequences on the OS and complicate the interpretation of the study results. Finally, there is no clear evidence that there are no biological differences between stages III and IV.

Age

Older age has been associated with a worse prognosis of PDAC, but it is not clear whether this is an effect related to the tumor, to the host, or to a lower prevalence of antineoplastic therapies (Aldoss 2011).

Of the 13 selected RCTs, 6 studied age in multivariate analysis: patients older than 65 years reported a poor prognosis in one study (Conroy 2011), while age was not associated with the outcome in the other 5 trials (Maisey 2002; Louvet 2005; Moore 2007; Poplin 2009; Colucci 2010).

In the PRODIGE4 study, however, there was a maximum limit of 75 years for enrollment, and also the effect of the experimental treatment arm was more relevant among elderly patients, suggesting a higher chemosensitivity, beyond the poor prognosis, for elderly patients (Conroy 2011). However, in a cohort study of 895 patients with mPDAC OS was reduced in patients more than 65 years old, but age did not change the prognosis among treated and untreated patients, while more elderly patients chose palliative therapies instead of cytotoxic chemotherapy (47% vs 25%), and 58% of those patients eligible for chemotherapy were not informed of their disease, so they could not make a treatment choice (Kuroda 2017).

Sex

Among the five studies of the 13 RCTs of mPDAC that evaluated this variable, only one study found an independent positive prognostic role for female sex (Moore 2007), while the other four did not document a significant relationship of sex with OS (Maisey 2002; Moore 2003; Poplin 2009; Colucci 2010).

Albumin

The role of albuminemia as PF is difficult to be assessed, given the close correlation between hypo-albuminemia and other variables associated with poor outcome, such as PS, older age, more advanced mPDAC, poor nutritional status, systemic inflammation, and hepatic dysfunction.

Among the 13 RCTs that reported a multivariate analysis, four included hypo-albuminemia, which predicted independently OS in two studies (Van Cutsem 2004; Conroy 2011), while in the other two it did not (Maisey 2002; Moore 2003).

Albuminemia is part of many prognostic scores, in particular in the modified Glasgow prognostic score (mGPS), which demonstrated prognostic value in PDAC in many series (Ahmad 2014). Furthermore, in studies of cytotoxic chemotherapy, hypo-albuminemia is expected to change the pharmacokinetics of antineoplastic drugs and consequently reduce their effectiveness. On the contrary, although the reasons are still unclear, a pooled analysis of seven prospective studies of mPDAC patients has documented that hypo-albuminemia could represent a predictor of efficacy of bevacizumab treatment, despite conditioning a greater elimination of bevacizumab; the analysis concluded that hypo-albuminemia was associated with a longer OS, and it was an independent PF in patients treated with bevacizumab, even after adjustment for PS and age (Pant 2014).

Tumor-Related Pain

Pain is a symptom that frequently accompanies the diagnosis of PDAC, so much so that it has also been used as one of the intermediate endpoints for the evaluation of the efficacy of antineoplastic medical therapies, such as the clinical benefit response, which allowed the registration of gemcitabine (Burris 1997; Colloca 2011). Advances in pain management, with improvements of regional and systemic treatments, have reduced its prevalence along the mPDAC course, weakening the predictive role of response to oncologic therapies but not the prognostic one.

Of the 13 selected RCTs, three included pain between the variables and all confirmed the independent relationship with the prognosis (Moore 2003; Van Cutsem 2004; Herrmann 2007).

Pain generation in PDAC appears to be a consequence of the presence of the phenomenon of perineural invasion by the tumor (Ceyhan 2010): by this mechanism neoplastic cells damage the myelin sheath of nerve cells (Di Mola 2008) and this event facilitates their proliferation and diffusion by neurotrophins and respective receptors, with the final activation of angiogenesis, which in turn increases pain. PDAC has the highest incidence of perineural invasion among all solid tumors, even in the early stages. A systematic review documented a poorer survival with the presence of perineural invasion in 11/13 studies, and in seven studies the association between perineural invasion and OS was significant. In fact, the median OS of patients with perineural invasion was lower, although not always significantly (Garcea 2008). In the future, it is therefore likely that pain may be an indicator of the PDAC sub-type and/or of specific activated signal pathways.

Pattern of Metastases

Characteristics of metastases have shown a correlation with patient survival in various tumors. In particular, in PDAC this association has been confirmed for the initial site of metastasis, it remains doubtful for the number of metastasis sites, whereas it needs more studies for timing.

Of the 13 selected RCTs, which reported a multivariate analysis, three documented a worse prognosis for patients with liver metastases (Oettle 2005; Conroy 2011; Von Hoff 2013). Indirectly, a similar situation can be inferred from two studies that, although they did not define the prognosis based on the site of metastases, found a shorter OS among cases with increased baseline serum levels of aspartate transaminase (AST) (Moore 2003) or alkaline phosphatase (ALP) (Maisey 2002). In a single study, the timing of metastases was investigated, and a poor OS emerged for patients with synchronous metastases compared to those with metachronous ones (Conroy 2011). In addition, also the number of metastatic sites was recently studied in two of the 13 RCTs, but the results were conflicting (Von Hoff 2013; Conroy 2011).

A SEER analysis of 13233 mPDAC patients diagnosed in 2010-2013 found that the outcome of patients with liver metastases was worse than that with distant lung or lymph node metastases (Oweira 2017). A study of 343 mPDAC patients focused on the presence at diagnosis of liver metastases only, extra-hepatic metastases or a combination of the two conditions. After multivariate analysis, the presence of hepatic metastases alone or in association with other sites, doubled the risk of death from mPDAC (HR 2.1-2.2), independently with respect to PS, albumin, and indexes of systemic inflammation (Kim 2015). Therefore, it has been hypothesized that the mPDAC with liver metastases is a biologically more aggressive disease, although from the studies on metachronous metastases two different phases were distinguished for the complex process of tumor metastasis to the liver, early dissemination and a later progression that followed the host immunosuppression (Shi 2016). The presence of extra-hepatic metastases compared to hepatic metastases alone further worsened the prognosis. In part this effect could be related to the presence of peritoneal metastases (Cao 2017; Morizane 2011), since peritoneal carcinomatosis remains more difficult to detect from radiology and is associated with shorter OS, both in a recent meta-analysis (Cao 2017) and from data of a cancer registry of 2924 PDAC (Thomassen 2013). In contrast to hepatic and peritoneal sites of metastasis, the presence of pulmonary metastases did not modify the prognosis in the PRODIGE4 study (Conroy 2011). Lung metastases, particularly metachronous, tend to be associated with a favorable course of mPDAC, with median OS up to 81.4 months (Lovececk 2017). Beyond the bias linked to the description of highly selected case reports or case studies, a subgroup of patients with only pulmonary metachronous recurrence, mainly women and with perineural invasion, has been described, and they showed a favorable trend of OS, so that it is suggested a regional treatment of isolated metachronous lung metastases (Decoster 2016; Zheng 2017). Very rare are the reports on bone metastases, which however are present in 5-20% of patients along the course of the disease (Hatfield 1976; Borad 2009). The prognosis of these patients is poor, although it correlates with PS, osteolysis, LDH, CRP, and inversely with time-to-bone metastasis (Outani 2018). Brain metastases are rare (0.2% of mPDAC) and late, usually following hepatic and pulmonary ones (Luu 2019), but also in these patients long-term survival is reported after resection (Lemke 2013).

Beyond the site, the unresectable disease often displays a different proliferative attitude, as demonstrated by the poor prognosis of synchronous metastases (Conroy 2011). The different molecular structures of the neoplasm and the response of the host could indeed generate completely different PDAC growth rates, regardless of the other variables. However, to date the evaluation of the growth rate of the mPDAC, even though it appears potentially relevant in clinical studies (Chiorean 2016; Robert 2017; Furukawa 2001; Mehrara 2009; Colloca 2016), has not been standardized or evaluated in large series.

Tumor Site (Head versus Body-Tail)

About 15-25% of PDACs arise in the pancreatic body or tail and their worst prognosis has often been attributed to a late presentation and diagnosis, characterized by weight loss and pain (Watanabe 2004). In reality, as far as the presentation stage is similar for head vs. body-tail PDACs (Sohn 2000), the literature reported conflicting conclusions on the site. PDACs of the head have a higher incidence, are easier to diagnose and have a better prognosis than those of body-tail (Ling 2013; Lau 2010), but survival is worse in localized cases (Lau 2010). According to other authors, the localization of PDAC at the head is associated with higher local invasiveness and relapsing capacity in seroso-cystic and intraductal papillary mucinous neoplasms (Khashab 2011; Park 2011). After one of the first reports about the different prognosis of the mPDACs arising in the two areas (Sohn 2000), a SEER analysis of 33752 PDAC patients at all stages documented the worst prognosis of body-tail tumors versus those of the head, with reduction of OS, increase in distant metastases, and reduction in the number of surgical procedures performed. In that SEER analysis, the relationship between site and prognosis was confirmed after multivariate analysis (Artinyan 2008).

Only two of the 13 selected RCTs analyzed the role of the primary tumor site, noting an independent relationship with the outcome in one study (Van

Cutsem 2004) but not in the other (Maisey 2002). In the PRODIGE-4 study, body-tail had worse survival after univariate analysis (Conroy 2011).

In addition to the different timing of symptoms onset, and therefore the possible later diagnosis for body-tail PDAC, it is necessary to consider the different embryological origin of the two areas, which arise from two distinct sites of the endoderm (Slack 1995), as well as the epidemiologic facts, reporting a 46% increase in incidence of body-tail PDACs in 30 years compared to a stable incidence of tumors of the pancreatic head (Lau 2010), all data that suggest a biological difference. In fact, an analysis of 521 patients of the Australian Pancreatic Cancer Genome (APGI) documented that the body-tail tumors presented a shorter survival than those of the head (12.1 vs 22.0 m), they were more often associated with the squamous molecular subtype, and displayed an activation of invasiveness pathways, of epithelial-mesenchymal transition program and a poor anti-tumor immune response. However, the authors were not able to establish if this correlated with a molecular characteristic or with a more advanced biological stage (Dreyer 2018).

Some data can be hypothesized for the primary site as a predictor of the efficacy of cytotoxic chemotherapy. Although the benefit from chemotherapy appears to be similar for all sites in mPDAC (Conroy 2011), a subgroup analysis of published studies raised doubts about the usefulness of gemcitabine-based adjuvant chemotherapy after resection of body-tail neoplasms, so the site has been proposed as a predictor of chemosensitivity (Mukhija 2018).

CA 19-9

Carbohydrate antigen 19-9 (CA 19-9) is a cell surface protein derived from the Lewis blood group antigen, expressed in 90-95% of the population, and overexpressed in 80% of the mPDACs (Boeck 2006). Some evidence supports a prognostic role for baseline CA 19-9 in mPDAC (Lim 2011; Tanaka 2008; Martin 2012; Koom 2009; An 2009, Yoo 2011), but there are many factors that can alter levels at diagnosis, including obstructive jaundice.

Three RCTs of the 13 previously selected evaluated baseline CA 19-9, and only one confirmed its independent prognostic value (Louvet 2005), while two more recent studies were negative (Conroy 2011; Von Hoff 2013).

Although in the MPACT study baseline CA 19-9 levels did not correlate with OS (Tabernero 2015), a subsequent analysis found a prognostic effect for CA 19-9 reduction after chemotherapy (Chiorean 2016), and a similar conclusion was reported in another analysis of the PRODIGE4 (Robert 2017). Although poorly studied in the context of RCTs, CA 19-9 kinetics after chemotherapy is an interesting variable, as documented by an individual patient data analysis of 6 studies of 212 mPDAC patients undergoing gemcitabine-based chemotherapy, which documented that the baseline value and the 5% increase after 2 cycles were associated with OS while the reduction after 2 cycles was not associated with the prognosis (Bauer 2013). Several small experiences have instead found a prognostic effect for CA 19-9 reduction after 8 weeks of chemotherapy (Halm 2000; Ko 2005; Hess 2008; Pelzer 2013), and for other CA 19-9 related tumor kinetic measures (Boeck 2010; Colloca 2016).

CEA

Carcinoembryonic antigen (CEA) is a complex glycoprotein of the membrane, which belongs to the immunoglobulin superfamily of cell adhesion molecules, also known as CEACAM5 or CD66e, which has a role in various cellular processes (Hammarstrom 1999). It is expressed by <50% of the cases with mPDAC.

Only one of the 13 RCT evaluated baseline CEA and documented an independent prognostic role (Conroy 2011).

Despite having been poorly studied in mPDAC, baseline CEA has been reported to be independent PF in several individual studies (Inal 2012; Lee 2013; Tsavaris 2009; Lee 2013; Reitz 2015; Wu 2015). From a biologic point of view, the CEA glycoprotein is a driver of tumor angiogenesis independent of the vascular endothelial growth factor (VEGF), and its expression could promote a tumor-favoring state of immunosuppression (Scurr 2015). It could, therefore, be a hallmark of the activation of a specific molecular pathway of mPDAC.

Weight Loss

Involuntary weight loss is one of the symptoms of the onset of PDAC and is associated with treatment failure. The cancer cachexia syndrome (CACS) is the most extreme consequence, defined as a complex metabolic derangement characterized by loss of muscle with or without the loss of fat, that cannot be reversed by nutritional support (Blum 2014). CACS is recognized as a major cause of decreased survival and treatment failure in patients with PDAC (Ozola Zalitel 2015), whereas weight stabilization is associated with improved OS (Davidson 2004). However, weight loss based on current criteria for CACS does not seem associated with a worse prognosis in PDAC patients (Nemer 2017). To date, studies on CACS in PDAC are limited, definitions are heterogeneous among studies, so even a recent meta-analysis was unable to determine the actual prognostic role of CACS and weight loss (Ozola Zalitel 2015).

Among the 13 selected RCTs that reported a multivariate analysis, only one evaluated weight loss and reported its correlation with OS (Van Cutsem 2004).

In another trial, weight loss was found to be significant in the univariate analysis only (Poplin 2009) and was not tested in multivariate. Although weight loss remains interesting as PF, its standard definition is complex and frequently retrospective, while prospective data on the role of CACS are necessary. Data from isolated studies suggest that different phenotypes of CACS in mPDAC patients receiving FOLFIRINOX may have different prognostic significance (Kays 2018). Sarcopenia, measured as skeletal muscle index or adipose tissue index, was an independent PF in patients with locally advanced PDAC receiving FOLFIRINOX chemotherapy, and was associated with increased myelotoxicity (Kurita 2019); similar results were reported after chemotherapy with gemcitabine (Park 2016).

Inflammation-Related Variables

Although there was no evidence from RCT, some other prognosis-related variables were considered relevant by experts, such as C-reactive protein, lactate dehydrogenase, the neutrophil-to-lymphocyte ratio (ter Veer 2018). This underlines how the activation of the inflammatory pathway by the PDAC is considered a very important step for prognostic purposes. However, there is still no standardized measurement to objectivate the phenomenon; on the contrary, many studies have evaluated single proteins, ratios, and scores. A list of the plethoric measurements of the activation of the systemic inflammatory response in patients with mPDAC is resumed in Table 2, but it is currently impossible to understand which are the most reliable variables. Single comparative experiences begin to be published, but evidence from RCTs, and their respective multivariate analyses are lacking.

The link between venous thromboembolism (VTE) and inflammation is widely documented in the literature, and in particular, among PDAC patients it is a negative prognostic variable, especially when occurring early or at diagnosis (Kim-2 2018). Among the predictors of thromboembolic risk in 168 patients with mPDAC, three emerged as independent (neutrophil-to-lymphocyte ratio, presence of the primary tumor, history of hypertension), suggesting that VTE is an epiphenomenon of the inflammatory state related to mPDAC (Mangla 2018). Although VTE has been reported as PF in univariate analysis in an RCT of patients with mPDAC receiving chemotherapy (Poplin 2009) it will be important to investigate in future RCTs on multivariate analysis. However, VTE is not even simple to objectivate due to a possible indolent clinical course, even though some authors suggest that it could be responsible for some early deaths in mPDAC patients, reducing the number of patients who receive chemotherapy or enter clinical trials (Fest 2017).

Table 2. Systemic inflammation-related variables, ratios, and scores predicting survival in studies of patients with unresectable or metastatic pancreatic adenocarcinoma

Variables

C-reactive protein (CRP)	(Szkandera 2014)
Lactate dehydrogenase (LDH)	(Yu 2017)
Leucocyte count	(Feng 2018)
Neutrophil count	(Feng 2018)
Neutrophil reduction	(Kurihara 2016)
Timing of neutropenia	(Chen 2017)

Ratios

Neutrophil-to-lymphocyte ratio (NLR)	(Xue 2014)
Derived neutrophil-to-lymphocyte ratio (dNLR)	(Suzuki 2015)
Platelet-to-lymphocyte ratio (PLR)	(Martin 2014)
Lymphocyte-to-monocyte ratio (LMR)	(Hu 2018)

Indexes

Prognostic Index	(Wang 2012)
Prognostic Nutritional Index	(Wang 2012)
Systemic-immuno-inflammation index (SIII)	(Aziz 2018)
Systemic inflammation response index (SIRI)	(Qi 2016)

Scores

Modified Glasgow Score (mGPS)	(Yamada 2016)
Neutrophil platelet score (NPS)	(Colloca 2018)
Tri-linear peripheric blood cell score (TRIS)	(Colloca 2018)

Prognostic Factors Combinations

Based on the prognostic factors summarized so far and others less studied, prognostic models (Yi 2011; Stocken 2008; Xue 2015; Forssell 2013), scores (Morizane 2011; Park 2016), and nomograms (Hang 2018) have been developed. The combination of PFs has often brought interesting results, frequently superior to the single variables, but the interpretation of the effectiveness of such tools is complex, both for the retrospective nature of the studies and for the treatments received from the patients, as well as for their limited replication in the literature.

Molecular Subtypes of PDAC

Since the intent of the current chapter is to resume published studies on PFs of mPDAC, which may be useful for clinicians, or to help them better understand the evolution of the knowledge of the disease, we have deliberately avoided reporting or attempting to summarize the large amount of molecular PFs, often reported in single studies including patients that have been poorly selected by stage and treatments. All these pieces of evidence, far from being uninteresting, seem inevitably to be part of a broader biological redefinition of PDAC that began from 2011, thanks to various genomic analyses, and in particular to the sequencing studies of RNA.

As in a giant puzzle, all these reports related to molecular markers with prognostic or predictive implications are intended to find their confirmation, but in the context of a phenotypic classification for PDAC subtypes. In fact, as for other neoplasms, a radical nosological revision seems to be emerging also for PDAC, which is likely to lead to a fragmentation in at least three different PDACs.

The most important studies about PDAC molecular classification are summarized in Table 3.

The first analysis of 27 cases allowed to define three subtypes of PDAC: classical, quasi-mesenchymal (QM-PDA) and exocrine-like (Collisson 2011). If the "classical" subtype has high expression of adhesion-associated and epithelial genes, the "QM-PDA" has a high expression of mesenchyme associated genes, while the "exocrine-like" displays relatively high levels of tumor cell-derived digestive enzyme genes.

Table 3. Proposed molecular classifications of pancreatic adenocarcinoma

Reference	
Collisson 2011	Materials: 27 tumor samples from resections performed at the University of California. Methods: gene expression analysis by non-negative matrix factorization with consensus clustering; definition of a 62 gene signature (PDAssigner). Results: detection of three subtypes (classical, quasi-mesenchymal, exocrine-like).
Moffitt 2015	Materials: 145 primary and 61 metastases of patients with pancreatic cancer. Methods: gene expression analysis by non-negative matrix factorization; validation on xenografts and cell cultures; analysis of gene expression from the stroma. Results: definition of a stromal classification (normal or activated) and four tumor-specific subtypes (classical, basal-like, exocrine pancreas factor, stromal).
Bailey 2016	Materials: 456 pancreatic tumors. Methods: identification of 32 recurrently mutated genes that aggregate into 10 pathways. Results: identification of four subtypes (squamous, pancreatic progenitor, immunogenic, aberrantly differentiated endocrine exocrine or ADEX).

This new variable, the molecular subtype, predicted the outcome independently with respect to the stage, with a better OS for the "classical" than the "QM-PDA". Furthermore, preclinical models, recreated for the first two molecular subtypes, allowed to observe a higher sensitivity to gemcitabine for "QM-PDA" compared to "classical", which however was more sensible to therapy with erlotinib, that appeared unusually more active in tumors with mutation of KRAS. Further studies are underway to develop simpler systems for defining the molecular subtype, such as the combination of GATA6 expression and KRAS status, which could soon identify the "classical" PDAC.

Another study included 145 PDACs and 61 metastases, and, in addition to making a decisive contribution to the molecular classification of PDAC, led to two important conclusions: the molecular characteristics of tumor and metastasis appear very similar in mPDAC; the characterization of the neoplastic stroma is essential to understanding the outcome of the tumor (Moffitt 2015). The stroma included 48% of the volume of the primitive tumor and was poorly represented in the metastasis, but worsened the outcome of the PDAC in which it was "activated", with the median OS that dropped from 24 to 15 months. Beyond the neoplastic cells, in fact, the activated stroma was richer in macrophage-associated genes, tumor-promoting genes, and fibroblast activating genes. In addition to stromal activation status, this classification distinguished two molecular subtypes of PDAC, "classical" and "basal-like", while two other subtypes (exocrine and stromal) were doubtful. The prognosis was very different between the two PDAC subtypes (median OS of 19 vs. 11 months) with almost all cases in stage IV classified as basal-like, which however expressed a better response to adjuvant chemotherapy with gemcitabine. After multivariate analysis, both classifications, stromal and PDAC cellular, were associated independently with OS. If there was a good genetic correspondence with the previous classification for the subgroups "classical" and "exocrine" with the correspondents of the Collisson classification, those of the subtype "QM-PDA" instead were included partly into the "basal-like" and partly into "stromal". KRAS mutations differed, with G12D overexpressed in the "basal-like" and G12V in "classical". The activation of the stroma also varied with the molecular subtype. In cell lines, basal-like PDACs had faster growth rates, which correlated with the worst prognosis. And even a clinical study, which stratified patients according to the Moffitt subtype, has documented better efficacy from chemotherapy in the "classical", in particular with FOLFIRINOX (Aung 2017).

Finally, a third molecular classification was reported by the APGI as part of the International Cancer Genome Consortium (ICGC) (Bailey 2016). This classification of PDAC was based on a huge number of molecular events (23538 mutations, 21208 genomic rearrangements, detected in 382 of the 456 cases) and defined four subtypes of PDAC (squamous; pancreatic progenitor; immunogenic; aberrantly differentiated endocrine or ADEX) discriminated by 10 different gene programs. Molecular subtypes expressed a relationship with specific histological features and everyone displayed its own specific transcriptional network. But only the "squamous" was independent PF.

Three of the four Bailey subtypes were similar to the corresponding Collisson ones, whereas the "immunogenic" was an exception. Thus, there was a similarity between subtypes, given that the "QM-PDA" corresponded to the "squamous", the "classical" to the "pancreatic progenitor", the "exocrine-like" to the "ADEX". One-half of Bailey's "squamous" tumors were part of the "basal-like" tumors by the Moffitt classification, while another half was a mixture of the other categories.

An analysis of 846 patients, after classifying their tumors according to these molecular classifications (Collisson, Moffitt tumor and stroma, Bailey), concluded that only the Bailey and the Moffitt stromal were associated with the outcome. Furthermore, all the classifications were associated with the pathological degree, and every tumor classification was able to predict a good or poor prognosis.

Real-time characterization of the mPDAC genome in the individual patient is now technically possible within the time of the clinical course of mPDAC, and sometimes it can guide clinical decision making or allow to enroll patients in clinical trials of personalized therapies (Aguirre 2018). This is thanks to the better definition of rapid strategies for defining the molecular subgroups (Muckenhuber 2018; Aung 2018).

Other classifications on chromosomal, mutational burden and epigenetic characteristics have been proposed, but they did not ever allow a prognostic correlation (Waddell 2015; Knudsen 2017; Mishra 2017; Lomberk 2018), although the role of methylation seems relevant (Nones 2014) as well as the characterization of some subgroups of the chromosomal classification (Waddell 2015).

Diagnostic Information for Patients with mPDAC

This process is essential to implement a new generation of clinical studies, since there is little correlation between the somatic mutational status of the most frequently mutated four genes of mPDAC (KRAS, TP53, SMAD4 and CDKN2A) and the efficacy of treatments (Gnant 2016; Qian 2018), due to the complex inter-relationships between oncogenesis drivers, signal pathway redundancy, bypass activation and other unknown molecular mechanisms (Singh 2019). The long series of failing studies of targeted therapies and immunotherapy in mPDAC is probably an effect of the complexity of the mechanisms of tumor progression, but it could be also linked to the lack of a molecular prognostic stratification of patients (Sheanan 2018).

Pending a comprehensive definition of the mPDAC subtypes, but also in order to contribute to their determination in the clinic and to understand the consequent changes in clinical practice, it is essential to guarantee the clinicians as much information as possible with respect to the individual patient. And at the moment in addition to the subtype, some features related to genetic mutations may have relevance for treatments. The finding of genomic alterations that can currently be targeted can only be done through a wide application of genetic tests, which until now have been limited to the subgroups of patients at risk for personal or family history. Nowadays, many of these tests are increasingly proposed as a routine examination in patients with PDAC (NCCN 3.2019).

Family history is an important risk factor for developing a PDAC. The definition of familial pancreatic cancer (FPC) refers to individuals with two or more first-degree relatives with PDAC (Petersen 2016), in which the known hereditary syndromes have been excluded (Steinberg 2009). Therefore, it is not surprising that similarly to other diseases, the number of affected family members increases the risk of PDAC, which ranges from 4.5 to 32 times, with one to three cases in the family (Klein 2004). More extensive studies document that a case of PDAC in a first-degree relative increases the risk by 1.8 times (Permuth-Wey 2009; Jacobs 2010). Whether, from a prognostic point of view, the neoplasms arising in FPC do not seem to differ from sporadic malignancies (Singhi 2015), the cases with FPC have allowed us to detect and characterize some germline mutations that guide the carcinogenesis of some PDACs.

In fact, hereditary PDAC is a heterogeneous entity, and could fall within the spectrum of some familial neoplastic syndromes, such as breast-ovarian cancer syndrome, Lynch syndrome, but also familial adenomatous polyposis, familial atypical multiple mole melanoma, Peutz-Jeghers syndrome, Li-Fraumeni syndrome, hereditary pancreatitis, von Hippel-Lindau syndrome and Fanconi syndrome (Ohmoto 2019; Slavin 2018). On the one hand, it must be considered that in the cases of family predisposition to PDAC the probability of detecting a mutated gene or a pathological polymorphism widening the genetic analysis could reach 30% of patients (Slavin 2018), even though genetic heterogeneity remains high. On the other hand, in the FPC kindreds, the proportion explained by germline mutations of known genetic syndromes remains too low, so low that even in a recent study the mutation rates were lower in the FPC probands than in the sporadic PDAC population (2.6% vs 4.0%) (Grant 2015). The variability of the patterns of the genes tested can partly explain these results, but the FPC is far from having been understood by the current discoveries, leaving to suspect that the bulk of the family predisposition is not linked to hereditary factors. Whether in more than 80% of the cases of FPC no known germline mutations are found, the known germinal alterations of hereditary PDAC are present in the sporadic PDAC at similar rates, so that many authors suggest to perform genetic diagnostic tests to all patients with PDAC diagnosis. In fact, a recent study (Hu 2018) on 3030 patients with PDAC and a considerable number of controls allowed to detect that in PDAC there is a mutation of one of 21 genes involved in genetic syndromes in 8.2%, in line with the literature (3.8-19.8%), often genes involved in DNA repair systems. In particular, there were 6 genes on which 5.5% of the cases detected were concentrated (ATM, BRCA1, BRCA2, CDKN2A, MLH1, TP53), which became 7.9% if patients were selected by family history. These patients had better OS (13.6 vs. 11.4 m; HR 0.86; 0.72-1.02), but the prognostic effect was not significant, as it was confirmed by another study on 615 patients with PDAC, which tested 76 gene panels, and reported a different but nonsignificant OS (50 vs. 34 m). The latter study detected pathogenetic germline alterations in 19.8% of patients, of which 41.8% would not have been never reported as the patients did not present the characteristics of eligibility for the genetic tests (Lowery 2018).

In the management of patients with an FPC, it is essential to proceed with the search for possible germline mutations with the purpose to obtain a diagnosis and genetic classification of the syndrome, but that information may have therapeutic implications (Lowery 2018; Klumpen 2011; Le 2018; Shindo 2017). A biomarker-driven strategy in drug selection could improve the outcome of patients with metastatic cancer, as reported by a systematic review that showed that 57% (21/37) of successful drug-programs adopted a biomarker-driven rationale compared to 16% (7/43) of failed drug-programs (Jardim 2017), but this is to be demonstrated in mPDAC patients. A recent systematic review identified 71 studies related to therapies driven by somatic or germline alterations, and concluded in favour of a wide analysis of germline mutations, reporting that in 36 studies the KRAS-pathway was affected with MEK-inhibitors, in other 22 the DNA homologous recombinant repair system was targeted with platinum salts and PARP-inhibitors and in other studies the MMR pathway with immunotherapy (Singh 2019).

Molecular Biology in the Clinical Management of mPDAC

The fact that the activated signal pathways are increasingly defined allows selecting subgroups of patients with mPDAC in which to test treatment strategies oriented by the biology of the disease. The reduction of the time necessary to test molecular diagnostics for biological characterization of the tumor has led to the conclusion that a large number of patients could be selected for targeted therapy, a proportion that should probably increase rapidly (Dreyer 2017).

Nevertheless, even in mPDAC management, the medical oncologist could draw some clinical indications from a wide biological characterization (Pihlak 2018).

BRCA Mutated mPDAC e BRCAness

Genomic instability detected by the Waddell classification co-segregated with inactivation of DNA repair/maintenance genes (BRCA1, BRCA2, PALB2) and a mutational signature of DNA damage repair deficiency (Waddell 2015). The alterations of the genes of this DNA repair system provide vulnerable targets for drugs such as platinum salts and PARP-inhibitors, which block the DNA single-strand break repair leading to double helix ruptures.

Pathogenetic germline mutations in BRCA genes and related genes are present in 4.6-8% of PDACs (The Cancer Genome Atlas Research Network 2017; Holter 2015; Salo-Mullen 2015). On the contrary, little is reported on the somatic mutations of these genes in the PDAC, which vary according to the study from 4 to 35% (Chantrill 2015; Witkiewicz 2015).

The dysfunction of the DNA repair system predicts a benefit of platinum salts similarly for germline and somatic mutations (Waddell 2015; Sehdev 2018). Platinum-based chemotherapy increased the median OS of 71 patients with a BRCA mutated mPDAC, from 9 to 22 months (Golan 2014), while in another study of 36 patients with a DDR-mutated mPDAC reported a marginal benefit in OS from FOLFIRINOX regimen, while the DDR-mutated status was associated with a better OS after multivariate analysis (Sehdev 2018). However, family history and personal history are insufficient criteria to select patients on platinum-based regimens, as documented in a study with GEMOX regimen (Takahashi 2018). PARP-inhibitors have been studied in BRCA-mutated mPDACs and in those with a BRCAness phenotype. However, even in these selected subgroups of patients they did not exceed 20-25% of overall response rate (Shroff 2018; De Bono 2017) and did not change the results of platinum-based chemotherapy, so much so that according to some authors, PARP-inhibitors should not be considered as an effective targeted therapy for PDACs with a BRCA signature (Pishvaian 2018). Preliminary data also suggest that BRCA signatures could correlate with a response to immunotherapy (Foley 2016).

Hyper-Mutated mPDAC

All of the hypermutated PDACs appear to be attributable to an MMR deficiency (Humphris 2017; Le 2017), even though a part of the hypermutated tumors is due to a smoke exposure signature and to previous treatment with alkylating agents (Campbell 2017). MMR-deficient tumors produce an increased amount of neo-antigens, which are associated with a higher rate of mutations, and a strong expression of ligands for checkpoint inhibitors (Le 2015). The frequency of MMR-deficient PDAC is around 1% of all PDAC.

Similarly to other tumors, immunotherapy with checkpoint inhibitors seems to prolong OS (Le 2015). Beyond the germinal mutations in genes of the MMR systems, even a reduction in the efficiency of the MMR system, such as MLH1 deficiency which has been documented in 9% of PDACs, could interfere with the response of mPDAC to treatments, as reported by an analysis of the RTOG 9704 trial (Lawrence 2018) and by the effect of polymorphisms on chemosensitivity (Dong 2009).

Immunogenic mPDAC (Bailey Classification)

Immunosuppression and the excessive role of the PDAC stroma are probably the major limits to a possible efficacy of immunotherapy, as it results from the complete lack of response to checkpoint inhibitors among patients with mPDAC without MMR deficit (Brahmer 2012). Although no study has been published about the activity of immunotherapy on the Bailey's "immunogenic" subtype of PDAC, this subtype has demonstrated upregulation of immune avoidance mechanisms, whereby various approaches are achieving interesting preliminary successes, such as the association of immunotherapy and chemotherapy after the inhibition of CXCR2 and FAK1, the CD40 stimulation (Steele 2016; Winograd 2015; Jiang 2016), the inhibition of the CCR3-CCL2 axis (Nywening 2016), and more generally the depletion of myeloid cells (Steele 2016; Nywening 2016; Zhang 2017).

ALK-Rearranged mPDAC

Although the translocation of ALK is rarely present in patients with PDAC (0.16%), as observed in a study of 3170 patients with only 5 rearrangements, its occurrence probability increases among subjects with <50 years (1.3%) (Singhi 2017).

In such PDACs, ALK inhibitors have been shown to be active.

CDK-Mutated mPDAC

Even though there are currently no active drugs present, new molecules may soon be associated to the inhibition of CDKN2A as well as CDK6, increasing the need for a molecular analysis extended to these genes (Ashgar 2015).

There are also two aspects of the pathogenesis of mPDAC, such as the role of angiogenesis and KRAS mutations, on which retrospective analyses of the previous negative RCTs would shed new light on the molecular landscape of mPDAC, beyond the reported failures.

PDAC is characterized by an intense inflammatory response (Hlatky 2002), it is a fibrotic and hypoxic tumor, extraordinarily rich in stroma, and producing high levels of pro-angiogenic molecules (Masamune 2010; Burris 1997), so much so that a prognostic role for many angiogenesis-related variables has been reported (Ikeda 1999; Seo 2000; Niedergethmann 2002; Erkan 2009; Kondo 2012). And some favorable clinical results have been shown by anti-angiogenic drugs in some minor studies (Reni 2013; Pant 2016; Martin 2012), so that a therapeutic role is advocated in association with new chemotherapy regimens, as a possible activity in avoiding the vascular rebound after tumor stromal reduction by nab-paclitaxel (von Hoff 2011; Seo 2000).

Activated KRAS occurs in 90-95% of PDAC, while NRAS and HRAS mutations are rare. The mutations are in the catalytic domain, they constitutionally activate the GTPase activity and the downstream pathway. These are early mutations, interesting G12 in 82% of tumors, and are insufficient for transformation. Although KRAS mutations are the most frequent in PDAC, there are no effective drugs for this target (Ostrem 2013; Patricelli 2016). Furthermore, striking downstream MEK was useless due to the reactivation of MAPK and collateral (Mai 2018), in particular, mediated by SHP2 and PTPN11, and little is known about the association antiMEK plus antiSHP2 combinations (Chen 2016). In addition, to date, it is not clear why the double inhibition (antiMEK + anti-EFGR) sometimes worked, while it has been useless to hit other pathway targets, such as PI3K and mTOR.

Conclusion

All the failing studies of targeted therapies remind us that we know little about the targets and the complex network of cellular and extracellular signals that drive the evolution and natural history of PDAC. However, such lack of knowledge leads us to a deep reflection on the meaning of what is a prognostic factor. This in fact, if on the one hand it is linked to the unitary definition of the mPDAC, which is now questioned by the molecular classification, on the other hand it is strongly linked to the "treatment arm" variable. The treatment arm could become increasingly complex, more like a global treatment strategy to address activated molecular pathways and individual tumor components (cell subgroups, stroma, etc). And when we think about the effects of drugs on tumor and stroma, our lack of knowledge expands, even whenever we discuss of cytotoxic chemotherapy.

The evolution of clinical trials is rapidly changing the reference prognostic variables, as it is happening for the PS in the case of non-cytotoxic medical therapies. Although every study will be designed to evaluate the "treatment arm" variable, it is not obvious that both the prognostic variables and the intermediate endpoints are adequate or that they will be in the future, as it has been just reported for traditional endpoints (Colloca 2016). It is therefore important to continue to include the "treatment arm" variable in the final prognostic model. This is because only the OS can sometimes allow us to evaluate the actual utility of a therapeutic procedure in medical oncology. Therefore, more than ever, the new therapies and the fragmentation of the nosological entity dramatically raise the problem of having reliable intermediate endpoints, a problem that is and will be the great challenge of clinical research in oncology. This applies to both regional and systemic treatments. For the latter, as we reported in the last part of this chapter, the endpoints will have to be drawn coherently with the molecular pathway and, as in other pathologies, the progressive prolongation of the median OS by treatments could change the reliable PFs and make very difficult to evaluate the effectiveness of first-line treatments. Therefore, it is inevitable that the panorama of prognostic and stratification factors will be changing towards molecular and less traditional variables, as has already begun (Aung 2017). On the other hand, PFs and endpoints of the studies are strongly connected, they depend on the clinical setting and on the type of therapy, and it is for this reason that new therapies in the more advanced phases of the mPDAC will be easily evaluated with old PFs and endpoint, like pain and clinical benefit response.

Finally, the complexity of cellular signals and the absence of any mPDAC with a single target to hit, substantiate the spectrum of a PDAC molecular evolution secondary to treatments, that could be different depending on its basic molecular structure (Mueller 2018). Little is known about this variable in a disease in which it has not yet been possible to hit one target successfully.

References

Aguirre, A.J., Nowak, J.A., Camarda, N.D., et al. "Real-time genomic characterization of advanced pancreatic cancer to enable precision medicine." *Cancer Discovery* 8, no. 9 (2018): 1096-111.

Ahmad, J., Grimes, N., Farid, S., et al. "Inflammatory response related scoring systems in assessing the prognosis of patients with pancreatic ductal adenocarcinoma: a systematic review." *Hepatobiliary & Pancreatic Diseases International* 13, no. 5 (2014): 474-81.

Aldoss, I.T., Tashi, T., Gonsalves, W., et al. "Role of chemotherapy in the very elderly patients with metastatic pancreatic cancer – A Veterans Affairs Cancer Registry analysis" *Journal of Geriatric Oncology* 2, no. 3 (2011): 209-14.

An, X., Li, Y.H., Lin, X.B., et al. "Prognostic value of serum CA 19-9 in patients with advanced pancreatic cancer receiving gemcitabine-based chemotherapy." *Chinese Journal of Cancer* 28, no. 3 (2009): 240-4.

Artinyan, A., Soriano, P.A., Prendergast, C., et al. "The anatomic location of pancreatic cancer is a prognostic factor for survival." *HPB* 10, no. 5 (2008): 371-6.

Ashgar, U., Witkiewicz, A.K., Turner, N.C., et al. "The history and future of targeting cyclin-dependent kinases in cancer therapy." *Nature Reviews. Drug Discovery* 14, no. 2 (2015): 130-46.

Atkinson, T.M., Andreotti, C.F., Roberts, K.E., et al. "The level of association between functional performance status measures and patient-reported outcomes in cancer patients: a systematic review." *Supportive Care in Cancer* 23, no. 12 (2015): 3645-52.

Aung, K.L., Fischer, S.E., Denroche, R.E., et al. "Genomics-driven precision medicine for advanced pancreatic cancer: early results from the COMPASS trial. *Clinical Cancer Research* 24, no. 6 (2018): 1344-54.

Aziz, M.H., Sideras, K., Aziz, N.A., et al. "The systemic-immune-inflammation index independently predicts survival and recurrence in resectable pancreatic cancer and its prognostic value depends on bilirubin levels. A retrospective multicenter cohort study. *Annals of*

Surgery (2018): doi: 10.1097/SLA.0000000000002660. [Epub ahead of print]

Bailey, P., Chang, D.K., Nones, K., et al. "Genomic analyses identify molecular subtypes of pancreatic cancer." *Nature* 531, no. 7592 (2016): 47-52.

Bauer, T.M., El-Rayes, B.F., Li, X., et al. "Carbohydrate antigen 19-9 is a prognostic and predictive biomarker in patients with advanced pancreatic cancer who receive gemcitabine-containing chemotherapy: a pooled analysis of 6 prospective trials." *Cancer* 119, vol. 2 (2013): 285-92.

Blum, D., Stene, G.B., Solheim, T.S., et al. "Validation of the Consensus-definition of cancer cachexia and evaluation of a classification model – a study based on data from an international multicentre project (EPCRC-CSA)." *Annals of Oncology* 25, no. 8 (2014): 1635-42.

Boeck, S., Haas, M., Laubender, R.P., et al. "Application of a time-varying covariate model to the analysis of CA 19-9 as serum biomarker in patients with advanced pancreatic cancer." *Clinical Cancer Research* 16, no. 3 (2010): 986-4.

Boeck, S., Stieber, P., Holdenrieder, S., et al. "Prognostic and therapeutic significance of carbohydrate antigen 19-9 as tumor marker in patients with pancreatic cancer." *Oncology* 70, no. 4 (2006): 255-64.

Borad, M.J., Saadati, H., Lakshmipathy, A., et al. "Skeletal metastases in pancreatic cancer: a retrospective study and review of the literature." *The Yale Journal of Biology and Medicine* 82, no. 1 (2009): 1-6.

Brahmer, J.R., Tykodi, S.S., Chow, L.Q., et al. "Safety and activity of anti-PD-L1 antibody in patients with advanced cancer." *New England Journal of Cancer* 366, no. 26 (2012): 2455 -65.

Burris, H.A., Moore, M.J., Andersen, J., et al. "Improvements in survival and clinical benefit with gemcitabine as first-line therapy for patients with advanced pancreas cancer: a randomized trial." *Journal of Clinical Oncology* 15, no. 6 (1997): 2403-13.

Campbell, B.B., Light, N., Fabrizio, D., et al. "Comprehensive analysis of hypermutation in human cancer." *Cell* 171, no. 5 (2017): 1042-56.

Cancer Stat Facts: Pancreatic Cancer. National Cancer Institute, accessed March 7, 2019, https://seer.cancer.gov/statfacts/html/pancreas.html.

Cao, F., Li, J., Li, A., et al. "Prognostic significance of positive peritoneal cytology in resectable pancreatic cancer: a systematic review and meta-analysis. *Oncotarget* 8, no. 9 (2017): 15004-13.

Ceyhan, G.O., Schafer, K.H., Kerscher, A.G., et al. "Nerve growth factor and artemin are paracrine mediators of pancreatic neuropathy in pancreatic adenocarcinoma." *Annals of Surgery* 251, no. 5 (2010); 923-31.

Chantrill, L.A., Nagrial, A.M., Watson, C., et al. "Precision medicine for advanced pancreas cancer: the individualized molecular pancreatic cancer therapy (IMPaCT) trial." *Clinical Cancer Research* 21, no. 9 (2015): 2029-37.

Chen, Y., Shi, Y., Yan, H., et al. "Timing of chemotherapy-induced neutropenia: the prognostic factor in advanced pancreatic cancer patients treated with gemcitabine / gemcitabine-based chemotherapy." *Oncotarget* 8, no. 39 (2017): 66593-600.

Chen, Y.N., LaMarche, M.J., Chan, H.M., et al. "Allosteric inhibition of SHP2 phosphatase inhibits cancers driven by receptor tyrosine kinases." *Nature* 535, no. 7610 (2016): 148-52.

Chiorean, E.G., Von Hoff, D., Wan, Y., et al. "Performance status dynamics during treatment with nab-paclitaxel plus gemcitabine versus gemcitabine alone for metastatic pancreatic cancer." *Cancer Management and Research* 10 (2018): 1389-96.

Chiorean, E.G., Von Hoff, D.D., Reni, M., et al. "CA 19-9 decrease at 8 weeks as a predictor of overall survival in a randomized phase III trial (MPACT) of weekly nab-paclitaxel plus gemcitabine versus gemcitabine alone in patients with metastatic pancreatic cancer" *Annals of Oncology* 27, no. 4 (2016): 654-60.

Collisson, E.A., Sadanandam, A., Olson, P., et al. "Subtypes of pancreatic ductal adenocarcinoma and their differing responses to therapy." *Nature Medicine* 17, no. 4 (2011): 500-3.

Colloca, G., Venturino, A., Guarneri, D. "Analysis of response-related and time-to-event endpoints in randomized trials of gemcitabine-based treatment versus gemcitabine alone as first-line treatment of patients with advanced pancreatic cancer." *Clinical Colorectal Cancer* 15, no. 3 (2016): 264-76.

Colloca, G., Venturino, A., Guarneri, D. "CA 19-9-related tumor kinetics after first-line chemotherapy of patients with advanced pancreatic cancer: a mono-institutional experience." *Medical Oncology* 33, no. 9 (2016): 103.

Colloca, G., Venturino, A. "Pain assessment in clinical trials of anticancer treatments." In *Horizons in Cancer Research*, Nova Publisher 2011; vol. 47(5).

Colloca, G.A., Venturino, A., Guarneri, D. "Second-generation inflammation-related scores are more effective than systemic inflammation ratios in predicting prognosis of patients with unresectable or metastatic pancreatic cancer receiving cytotoxic chemotherapy." *Medical Oncology* 35, no. 12 (2018): 158.

Colucci, G., Labianca, R., Di Costanzo, F., et al. "Randomized phase III trial of gemcitabine plus cisplatin compared with single-agent gemcitabine as first-line treatment of patients with advanced pancreatic cancer: the GIP-1 study." *Journal of Clinical Oncology* 28, no. 10 (2010): 1645-51.

Conroy, T., Desseigne, F., Ychou, M., et al. "FOLFIRINOX versus gemcitabine for metastatic pancreatic cancer." *New England Journal of Medicine* 364, no. 19 (2011): 1817-25.

Conroy, T., Hammel, P., Hebbar, M., et al. "FOLFIRINOX or gemcitabine as adjuvant therapy for pancreatic cancer." *New England Journal of Medicine* 379, no. 25 (2018): 2395-406.

Davidson, W., Ash, S., Capra, S., et al. "Weight stabilisation is associated with improved survival duration and quality of life in unresectable pancreatic cancer." *Clinical Nutrition* 23, no. 2 (2004): 239-47.

de Bono, J., Ramanathan, R.K., Mina, L., et al. "Phase I, dose-escalation, two-part trial of the PARP inhibitor talazoparib in patients with advanced germline BRCA1/2 mutations and selected sporadic cancers." *Cancer Discovery* 7, no. 6 (2017): 620-9.

Decoster, C., Gilabert, M., Autret, A., et al. "Heterogeneity of metastatic pancreatic adenocarcinoma: lung metastasis show better prognosis than liver metastasis – a case control study." *Oncotarget* 7, no. 29 (2016): 45649-55.

di Mola, F.F., di Sebastiano, P. "Pain and pain generation in pancreatic cancer." *Langenbeck's Archives of Surgery* 393, vol. 6 (2008): 919-22.

Dong, X., Jiao L, Li Y, et al. "Significant association of mismatch repair gene polymorphisms with clinical outcome of pancreatic cancer." *Journal of Clinical Oncology* 27, no. 10 (2009): 1592-9.

Dreyer, S.B., Chang, D.K., Bailey, P., et al. "Pancreatic cancer genomes: implications for clinical management and therapeutic development." *Clinical Cancer Research* 23, no. 7 (2017): 1638-46.

Dreyer, S.B., Jamieson, N.B., Upstill-Goddard, R., et al. "Defining the molecular pathology of pancreatic body and tail adenocarcinoma." *British Journal of Surgery* 105: no. 2 (2018): e183-91.

Ducreux, M., Rougier, P., Pignon, J.-P., et al. "A randomised trial comparing 5-FU with 5-FU plus cisplatin in advanced pancreatic carcinoma." *Annals of Oncology* 13, no. 8 (2002): 1185-91.

Erkan, M., Reiser-Erkan, C., Michalski, C.W., et al. "Cancer-stellate cell interactions perpetuate the hypoxia-fibrosis cycle in pancreatic ductal adenocarcinoma." *Neoplasia* 11, no. 5 (2009): 497-508.

Feng, L., Gu, S., Wang, P., et al. "White blood cell and granulocyte counts are independent predictive factors for prognosis of advanced pancreatic cancer." *Gastroenterology Research and Practice* (2018): 8096234.

Ferlay, J., Partensky, C., and Bray, F. "More deaths from pancreatic cancer than breast cancer in the EU by 2017." *Acta Oncologica* 55, no. 9-10 (2016): 1158-60.

Fest, J., Ruiter, R., van Rooij. F.J.A., et al. "Underestimation of pancreatic cancer in the national cancer registry - Reconsidering the incidence and survival rates." *European Journal of Cancer* 72, no. (2017): 186-91.

Foley, K., Kim, V., Jaffee, E., et al. "Current progress in immunotherapy for pancreatic cancer." *Cancer Letters* 381, no. 1 (2016): 244-51.

Forssell, H., Wester, M., Akesson, K, et al. "A proposed model for prediction of survival based on a follow-up study in unresectable pancreatic cancer." *BMJ Open* 3 (2013): e004064.

Furukawa, H., Iwata, R., Moriyama, N. "Growth rate of pancreatic adenocarcinoma: initial clinical experience." *Pancreas* 22, no. 4 (2001): 366-9.

Garcea, G., Dennison, A.R., Pattenden, C.J., et al. "Survival following curative resection for pancreatic ductal adenocarcinoma. A systematic review of the literature." JOP: *Journal of the Pancreas* 9, vol. 2 (2008): 99-132.

Gnant, T.J., Hua, K., Singh, A. "Molecular pathogenesis of pancreatic cancer." *Progress in Molecular Biology and Translational Science* 144, no. (2016): 241-75.

Golan, T., Kanji, Z.S., Epelbaum, R., et al. "Overall survival and clinical characteristics of pancreatic cancer in BRCA mutation carriers." *British Journal of Cancer* 111, no. 6 (2014): 1132-8.

Grant, R.C., Selander, I., Connor, A.A., et al. "Prevalence of germline mutations in cancer predisposition genes in patients with pancreatic cancer." *Gastroenterology* 148, no. 3 (2015): 556-64.

Halm, U., Schumann, T., Schiefke, I., et al. "Decrease of CA 19-9 during chemotherapy with gemcitabine predicts survival time in patients with advanced pancreatic cancer." *British Journal of Cancer* 82, no. 5: 1013-6.

Hammarstrom, S. "The carcinoembryonic antigen (CEA) family: structures, suggested functions and expression in normal and malignant tissues." *Seminars in Cancer Biology* 9, no. 2 (1999): 67-81.

Hammel, P., Huguet, F., van Laethem, J.-L., et al. "Effect of chemoradiotherapy vs chemotherapy on survival in patients with locally advanced pancreatic cancer controlled after 4 months of gemcitabine with or without erlotinib. The LAP07 randomized clinical trial." *Journal of the American Medical Association* 315, no. 17 (2016): 1844-53.

Hang, J., Wu, L., Zhu, L., et al. "Prediction of overall survival for metastatic pancreatic cancer: development and validation of a prognostic nomogram with data from open clinical trial and real-world study." *Cancer Medicine* 7 (2018): 2974-84.

Hatfield, D.R., DeLand, F.H., Maruyama, Y. "Skeletal metastases in pancreatic carcinoma: study by isotopic bone scanning." *Oncology* 33, no. 1 (1976): 44-7.

Herrmann, R., Bodoky, G., Rushstaller, T., et al. "Gemcitabine plus capecitabine compared with gemcitabine alone in advanced pancreatic cancer: a randomized, multicenter, phase III trial of the Swiss Group for Clinical Cancer Research and the Central European Cooperative Oncology Group." *Journal of Clinical Oncology* 25, no. 16 (2007): 2212-7.

Hess, V., Glimelius, B., Grawe, P., et al. "CA 19-9 tumor marker response to chemotherapy in patients with advanced pancreatic cancer enrolled in a randomised controlled trial." *Lancet Oncology* 9, no. 2 (2008): 132-8.

Hlatky, L., Hahnfeldt, P., Folkman, J. "Clinical application of antiangiogenetic therapy: microvessel density, what it does and doesn't tell us." *Journal of the National Cancer Institute* 94, no. 12 (2002): 883-93.

Holter, S., Borgida, A., Dodd, A., et al. "Germline BRCA mutations in a large clinic-based cohort of patients with pancreatic adenocarcinoma." *Journal of Clinical Oncology* 33, no. 28 (2015): 3124-9.

Hu, R.J., Ma, J.Y., Hu, G. "Lymphocyte-to-monocyte ratio in pancreatic cancer: prognostic significance and meta-analysis." *Clinica Chimica Acta* 481 (2018): 142-6.

Hu, Z.I., Shia, J., Stadler, Z.K., et al. "Evaluating mismatch repair deficiency in pancreatic adenocarcinoma: challenges and recommendations." *Clinical Cancer Research* 24, no. 6 (2018): 1326-36.

Humphris, J.L., Patch, A.M., Nones, K., et al. "Hypermutation in pancreatic cancer." *Gastroenterology* 152, no. 1 (2017): 68-74.

Ikeda, N., Adachi, M., Taki, T., et al. "Prognostic significance of angiogenesis in human pancreatic cancer." *British Journal of Cancer* 79, no. 0-10 (1999): 1553-63.

Inal, A., Kos, F.T., Algin, E., et al. "Prognostic factors in patients with advanced pancreatic cancer treated with gemcitabine alone or gemcitabine plus cisplatin: retrospective analysis of a multicenter study." *Journal of the Balkan Union of Oncology* 17, no. 1 (2012): 102-5.

Inoue, A., Kobayashi, K., Usui, K., et al. "First-line gefitinib for patients with advanced non-small-cell lung cancer harboring epidermal growth factor receptor mutations without indication for chemotherapy." *Journal of Clinical Oncology* 27, no. 9 (2009): 1394-400.

Jardim, D.L., Groves, E.S., Breitfeld, P.P., et al. "Factors associated with failure of oncology drugs in late-stage clinical development: a systematic review." *Cancer Treatment Reviews* 52, no. 1 (2017): 12-21.

Jiang, H., Hedge, S., Knolhoff, B.L., et al. "Targeting focal adhesion kinase renders pancreatic cancers responsive to checkpoint immunotherapy." *Nature Medicine* 22, no. 8 (2016): 851-60.

Kadokura, M., Ishida, Y., Tatsumi, A., et al. "Performance status and neutrophil-lymphocyte ratio are important prognostic factors in elderly patients with unresectable pancreatic cancer." *Journal of Gastrointestinal Oncology* 7, no. 6 (2016): 982-8.

Karnofsky, D.A. and Burchenal, J.H. "The clinical evaluatuion of chemotherapeutic agents in cancer," in MacLeod C (ed): *Evaluation of Chemotherapeutic Agents*. New York, NY, Columbia University Press, 1949, pp 191-205.

Katz, M.H., Wang, H., Fleming, J.B., et al. "Long-term survival after multidisciplinary management of resected pancreatic adenocarcinoma." *Annals of Surgical Oncology* 16, no. 4 (2009): 836-47.

Kays, J.K., Shahda, S., Stanley, M., et al. "Three cachexia phenotypes and the impact of fat-only loss on survival in FOLFIRINOX therapy for pancreatic cancer." *Journal of Cachexia, Sarcopenia and Muscle* 9, no. 4 (2018): 673-84.

Khashab, M.A., Shin, E.J., Amateau, S., et al. "Tumor size and location correlate with behaviour of pancreatic serous cystic neoplasms." *American Journal of Gastroenterology* 106, no. 8 (2011): 1521-6.

Kim, H.W., Lee, J.-C., Paik, K.-H., et al. "Initial metastatic site as a prognostic factor in patients with stage IV pancreatic ductal adenocarcinoma." *Medicine* 94, no. 25 (2015): e1012.

Kim, J.S., Kang, E.J., Kim, D.S., et al. "Early venous thromboembolism at the beginning of palliative chemotherapy is a poor prognostic factor in patients with metastatic pancreatic cancer: a retrospective study." *BMC Cancer* 18 (2018): 1260.

Kindler, H.L., Ioka, T., Richel, D., et al. "Axitinib plus gemcitabine versus placebo plus gemcitabine in patients with advanced pancreatic adenocarcinoma: a double-blind randomised phase 3 study." *Lancet Oncology* 12, no. 3 (2011): 256-62.

Klein, A.P., Brune, K.A., Petersen, G.M., et al. "Prospective risk of pancreatic cancer in familial pancreatic cancer kindreds." *Cancer Research* 64, no. 7 (2004): 2634-8.

Klumpen, H.-J., Queiroz, K.C.S., Spek, C.A., et al. "mTOR inhibitor treatment of pancreatic cancer in a patient with Peutz-Jegher syndrome." *Journal of Clinical Oncology* 29, no. 6 (2011): e150-3.

Knudsen, E.S., Vail, P., Balaji, U., et al. "Stratification of pancreatic ductal adenocarcinoma: combinatorial genetic, stromal, and immunologic markers." *Clinical Cancer Research* 23, no. 15 (2017): 4429-40.

Ko, A.H., Hwang, J., Venook, A.P., et al. "Serum CA 19-9 response as a surrogate for clinical outcome in patients receiving fixed-dose rate gemcitabine for advanced pancreatic cancer." *British Journal of Cancer* 93, no. 2 (2005): 195-9.

Kondo, S., Ueno, H., Hashimoto, J., et al. "Circulating endothelial cells and other angiogenesis factors in pancreatic carcinoma patients receiving gemcitabine chemotherapy." *BMC Cancer* 12 (2012): 268.

Koom, W.S., Seong, J., Kim, Y.B., et al. "CA 19-9 as a predictor for response and survival in advanced pancreatic cancer patients treated with chemoradiotherapy." *International Journal of Radiation Oncology Biology Physics* 73, no. 4 (2009): 1148-54.

Kurihara, T., Kogo, M., Ishii, M., et al. "Chemotherapy-induced neutropenia as a prognostic factor in patients with unresectable pancreatic cancer." *Cancer Chemother Pharmacol* 76, no. 6 (2015): 1217-24.

Kurita, Y., Kobayashi, N., Tokuhisa, M., et al. "Sarcopenia is a reliable prognostic factor in patients with advanced pancreatic cancer receiving FOLFIRINOX chemotherapy." *Pancreatology* 19, no. 1 (2019): 127-35.

Kuroda, T., Kumagi, T., Yokota, T., et al. "Efficacy of chemotherapy in elderly patients with unresectable pancreatic cancer: a multicenter review of 895 patients." *BMC Gastroenterology* 17 (2017): 66.

Laird, B.J.A., Fallon, M., Hjermstad, M.J., et al. "Quality of life in patients with advanced cancer: differential association with performance status and systemic inflammatory response." *Journal of Clinical Oncology* 34, no. 23 (2016): 2769-75.

Langer, C.J. "The Lazarus response in treatment-naive, poor performance status patients with non-small-cell lung cancer and epidermal growth factor receptor mutation." *Journal of Clinical Oncology* 27, no. 9 (2009): 1350-4.

Lau, M.K., Davila, J.A., Shaib, Y.H. "Incidence and survival of pancreatic head and body and tail cancers: a population-based study in the United States." *Pancreas* 39, no. 4 (2010): 458-62.

Lawrence, Y.R., Moughan, J., Magliocco, A.M., et al. "Expression of the DNA repair gene MLH1 correlates with survival in patients who have resected pancreatic cancer and have received adjuvant chemoradiation: NRG Oncology RTOG study 9704." *Cancer* 124, no. 3 (2018): 491-8.

Le, D.T., Durham, J.N., Smith, K.N., et al. Mismatch repair deficiency predicts response of solid tumors to PD-1 blockade." *Science* 357, no. 6349 (2017): 409-13.

Le, D.T., Uram, J.N., Wang, H., et al. "PD-1 blockade in tumors with mismatch-repair deficiency." *New England Journal of Medicine* 372, no. 26 (2015): 2509-20.

Lee, K.J., Li, S.W., Chung, M.J., et al. "Serum CA 19-9 and CEA levels as a prognostic factor in pancreatic adenocarcinoma." *Yonsei Medical Journal* 54, no. 3 (2013): 643-9.

Lemke, J., Scheele, J., Kappa, T., et al. "Brain metastasis in pancreatic cancer." *International Journal of Moleclar Sciences* 14, no. 2 (2013): 4163-73.

Li, D., Xie, K., Wolff, R., et al. "Pancreatic cancer." *Lancet* 363, no. 9414 (2004): 1049-57.

Lim, K.H., Kim, T.Y., Lee, K.H., et al. "Efficacy of infusional 5-fluorouracil, doxorubicin, and mitomycin-C (FAM) in the treatment of patients with gemcitabine-pretreated pancreatic cancer and analysis of prognostic factors in a salvage setting." *Cancer Chemotherapy and Pharmacology* 68, no. 4 (2011): 1017-26.

Ling, Q., Xu, X., Zheng, S.S., et al. "The diversity between pancreatic head and body/tail cancers: clinical parameters and in vitro models." *Hepatobiliary & Pancreatic Diseases International* 12, no. 5 (2013): 480-7.

Lomberk, G., Blum, Y., Nicolle, R., et al. "Distinct epigenetic landscapes underlie the pathobiology of pancreatic cancer subtypes." *Nature Communications* 9 (2018): 1978.

Louvet, C., Labianca, R., Hammel, P., et al. "Gemcitabine in combination with oxaliplatin compared with gemcitabine alone in locally advanced or metastatic pancreatic cancer: results of a GERCOR and GISCAD phase III trial." *Journal of Clinical Oncology* 23, no. 15 (2005): 3509-16.

Lovececk, M., Skalicky, P., Chudacek, J., et al. "Different clinical presentations of metachronous pulmonary metastases after resection of pancreatic ductal adenocarcinoma: retrospective study and review of the literature." *World Journal of Gastroenterology* 23, no. 35 (2017): 6420-8.

Lowery, M.A., Kelsen, D.P., Capanu, M., et al. "Phase II trial of veliparib in patients with previously treated BRCA-mutated pancreas ductal adenocarcinoma." *European Journal of Cancer* 89 (2018): 19-26.

Lowery, M.A., Wong, W., Jordan, E.J., et al. "Prospective evaluation of germline alterations in patients with exocrine pancreatic neoplasms." *Journal of the National Cancer Institute* 110, no. 10 (2018): djy024.

Luu, A.M., Kunzli, B., Hoehn, P., et al. "Prognostic value and impact of cerebral metastases in pancreatic cancer." *Acta Chirurgica Belgica* (2019): doi: 10.1080/00015458.2018 [Epub ahead of print]

Mai, T.T. and Lito, P. "A treatment strategy for KRAS-driven tumors." *Nature Medicine* 24, no. 7 (2018): 902-4.

Maisey, N., Chau, I., Cunningham, D., et al. "Multicenter randomized phase III trial comparing protracted venous infusion (PVI) fluorouracil (5-FU) with PVI 5-FU plus mitomycin in inoperable pancreatic cancer." *Journal of Clinical Oncology* 20, no. 14 (2002): 3130-6.

Mangla, A., Mushtaq, M.U., Agarwal, N., et al. "Retrospective analysis of factors associated with venous thromboembolism among pancreatic cancer patients. A single institution experience." *Pancreas* 47, no. 8 (2018): e52-3.

Martin, H.L., Ohara, K., Kiberu, A., et al. "Prognostic value of systemic inflammation-based markers in advanced pancreatic cancer." *Internal Medicine Journal* 44, no. 7 (2014): 676-82.

Martin, L.K. "Elevated baseline CA 19-9 levels correlate with adverse prognosis in patients with early- or advanced-stage pancreas cancer." *Medical Oncology* 29, no. 5 (2012): 3101-7.

Masamune, A., Watanabe, T., Kikuta, K., et al. "Nuclear expression of interleukin-33 in pancreatic stellate cells." *American Journal of Physiology. Gastrointestinal and Liver Physiology* 295, no. 4 (2010): G821-32.

Mehrara, E., Forssell-Aronsson, E., Ahlman, H., et al. "Quantitative analysis of tumor growth rate and changes in tumor marker level: specific growth rate versus doubling time." *Acta Oncologica* 48, no. 4 (2009): 591-7.

Mishra, N.K., Guda, C. "Genome-wide DNA methylation analysis reveals molecular subtypes of pancreatic cancer." *Oncotarget* 8, no. 17 (2017): 28990-9012.

Moffitt, R.A., Marayati, R., Flate, E.L., et al. Virtual microdissection identifies distinct tumor- and stroma-specific subtypes of pancreatic ductal adenocarcinoma. *Nature Genetics* 47, no. 10 (2015): 1168-78.

Moore, M.J., Goldstein, D., Hamm, J., et al. "Erlotinib plus gemcitabine compared with gemcitabine alone in patients with advanced pancreatic cancer: a phase III trial of the National Cancer Institute of Canada Clinical Trials Group." *Journal of Clinical Oncology* 25, no. 15 (2007): 1960-6.

Moore, M.J., Hamm, J., Dancey, J., et al. "Comparison of gemcitabine versus the matrix metalloproteinase inhibitor BAY 12-9566 in patients with advanced or metastatic adenocarcinoma of the pancreas: a phase III trial of the National Cancer Institute of Canada Clinical Trials Group." *Journal of Clinical Oncology* 21, no. 17 (2003): 3296-302.

Morizane, C., Okusaka, T., Morita, S., et al. "Construction and validation of a prognostic index for patients with metastatic pancreatic adenocarcinoma." *Pancreas* 40, no. 3 (2011): 415-21.

Muckenhuber, A., Berger, A.K., Schilitter, A.M., et al. "Pancreatic ductal adenocarcinoma subtyping using the biomarkers hepatocyte nuclear factor-1A and cytokeratin-81 correlates with outcome and treatment response." *Clinical Cancer Research* 24, no. 2 (2018): 351-9.

Mueller, S., Engleitner, T., Maresch, R., et al. "Evolutionary routes and KRAS dosage define pancreatic cancer phenotypes." *Nature* 554, n. 7690 (2018): 62-8.

Mukhija, D., Sohal, D.P.S., Khorana, A.A. "Adjuvant treatment in potentially curable pancreatic cancer need to include tumor location in the equation?" *Pancreas* 47, n. 8 (2018): e50-2.

NCCN clinical practice guidelines in oncology. *Genetic/familial high-risk assessment: breast and ovarian* - version 3.2019, accessed May 2, 2019, https://www.nccn.org/professionals/physician_gls/pdf/genetics_screening.pdf.

Nemer, L., Krishna, S.G., Shah, Z.K., et al. "Predictors of pancreatic cancer-associated weight loss and nutritional interventions." *Pancreas* 46, no. 9 (2017): 1152-7.

Niedergethmann, M., Hildenbrand. R., Wostbrock, B., et al. "High expression of vascular endothelial growth factor predicts early recurrence and poor prognosis after curative resection for ductal adenocarcinoma of the pancreas." *Pancreas* 25, no. 2 (2002): 122-9.

Nones, K., Waddell, N., Song, S., et al. "Genome-wide DNA methylation patterns in pancreatic ductal adenocarcinoma reveal epigenetic deregulation of SLIT-ROBO, ITGA2 and MET signaling." *International Journal of Cancer* 135, no. (2014): 1110-8.

Nywening, T.M., Wang-Gillam, A., Sanford, D.E., et al. "Targeting tumour-associated macrophages with CCR2 inhibition in combination with FOLFIRINOX in patients with borderline resectable and locally advanced pancreatic cancer: a single-center, open-label, dose-finding, non-randomised, phase 1b trial." *Lancet Oncology* 17; no. 5 (2016): 651-62.

Oettle, H., Richards, D., Ramanathan, R.K., et al. "A phase III trial of pemetrexed plus gemcitabine versus gemcitabine in patients with unresectable or metastatic pancreatic cancer." *Annals of Oncology* 16, no. 10 (2005): 1639-45.

Ohmoto, A., Yachida, S., Morizane, C. "Genomic features and clinical management of patients with hereditary pancreatic cancer syndromes and familial pancreatic cancer." *International Journal of Molecular Sciences* 20, no. (2019): 561.

Oken, M.M., Creech, R.H., Tormey, D.C., et al. "Toxicity and response criteria of the Eastern Cooperative Oncology Group." *American Journal of Clinical Oncology* 5, no. 6, (1982): 649-55.

Ostrem, J.M., Peters, U., Sos, M.L., et al. "K-Ras(G12C) inhibitors allosterically control GTP affinity and effector interactions." *Nature* 503, no. 7477 (2013): 548-51.

Outani, H., Akita, H., Nakai, T., et al. "Clinical features and prognosis of patients with the bone metastasis of pancreatic cancer. A single-institutional cohort study." *Pancreas* 47, no. 7 (2018): e43-6.

Oweira, H., Petrausch, U., Helbling, D., et al. "Prognostic value of site-specific metastases in pancreatic adenocarcinoma: a Surveillance Epidemiology and End Results database analysis." *World Journal of Gastroenterology* 23, no. 10 (2017): 1872-80.

Ozola Zalitel, I., Zykus, R., Francisco Gonzalez, M., et al. "Influence of cachexia and sarcopenia on survival in pancreatic ductal adenocarcinoma: a systematic review." *Pancreatology* 15, no. 1 (2015): 19-24.

Pant, S., Martin, L.K., Geyer, S., et al. "Baseline serum albumin is a predictive biomarker for patients with advanced pancreatic cancer treated with bevacizumab: a pooled analysis of 7 prospective trials of gemcitabine-based therapy with or without bevacizumab." *Cancer* 120, no. 12 (2014): 1780-6.

Pant, S., Martin, L.K., Geyer, S., et al. "Treatment-related hypertension as a pharmacodynamic biomarker for the efficacy of bevacizumab in advanced pancreas cancer. A pooled analysis of 4 prospective trials of gemcitabine-based therapy with bevacizumab." *American Journal of Clinical Oncology* 39, no. 6 (2016): 614-8.

Park, I., Choi, S.J., Kim, Y.S., et al. "Prognostic factors for risk stratification of patients with recurrent or metastatic pancreatic adenocarcinoma who were treated with gemcitabine-based chemotherapy." *Cancer Research and Treatment* 48 (2016): 1264-73.

Park, J., Lee, K.T., Jang, T.H., et al. "Risk factors associated with the postoperative recurrence of intraductal papillary mucinous neoplasms of the pancreas." *Pancreas* 40, no. 1 (2011): 46-51.

Patricelli, M.P., Janes, M.R., Li, L.S., et al. "Selective inhibition of oncogenic KRAS output with small molecules targeting the inactive state." *Cancer Discovery* 6, no. 3 (2016): 316-29.

Pelzer, U., Hilbig, A., Sinn, M., et al. "Value of carbohydrate antigen 19-9 in predicting response and therapy control in patients with metastatic pancreatic cancer underoing first-line therapy." *Frontiers in Oncology* 3 (2013): 155.

Permuth-Wey, J., and Egan, K.M. "Family history is a significant risk factor for pancreatic cancer: results from a systematic review and meta-analysis." *Familial Cancer* 8, no. 2 (2009): 109-17.

Petersen, G.M. "Familial pancreatic cancer." *Seminars in Oncology* 43, no. 5 (2016): 548-53.

Pihlak, R., Weaver, J.M.J., Valle, J.W., et al. "Advances in molecular profiling and categorisation of pancreatic adenocarcinoma and the implications for therapy." *Cancers* 10 (2018): 17.

Pishvaian, M.J., Petricoin, E. "Molecular profiling of pancreatic cancer patients – response." *Clinical Cancer Research* 24, no. 24 (2018): 2211-2.

Poplin, E., Feng, Y., Berlin, J., et al. "Phase III, randomized study of gemcitabine and oxaliplatin versus gemcitabine (fixed-dose rate infusion) compared with gemcitabine (30-minute infusion) in patients with pancreatic carcinoma E6201: a trial of the Eastern Cooperative Oncology Group." *Journal of Clinical Oncology* 27, no. 23 (2009): 3778-85.

Qi, Q., Zhuang, L., Shen, Y., et al. A novel systemic inflammation response index (SIRI) for predicting the survival of patients with pancreatic cancer after chemotherapy. *Cancer* 122, no. 14 (2016): 2158-67.

Qian, Z.R., Rubinson, D.A., Nowak, J.A., et al. "Association of alterations in main driver genes with outcomes of patients with resected pancreatic ductal adenocarcinoma." *JAMA Oncology* 4, no. 3 (2018): e173420.

Rawla, P., Sunkara, T., Gaduputi, V. "Epidemiology of pancreatic cancer: global trends, etiology and risk factors." *World Journal of Oncology* 10, no. 1 (2019): 10-27.

Reitz, D., Gerger, A., Seidel, J., et al. "Combination of tumour markers CEA and CA 19-9 improves the prognostic prediction in patients with pancreatic cancer." *Journal of Clinical Pathology* 68, no. 6 (2015): 427-33.

Reni, M., Cereda, S., Milella, M., et al. "Maintenance sunitinib or observation in metastatic pancreatic adenocarcinoma: a phase II randomised trial." *European Journal of Cancer* 49, no. 17 (2013): 3609-15.

Robert, M., Jarlier, M., Gourgou, S., et al. "Retrospective analysis of CA 19-9 decrease in patients with metastatic pancreatic carcinoma treated with FOLFIRINOX or gemcitabine in a randomized phase III study (ACCORD11/PRODIGE4)." *Oncology* 93, no. 6 (2017): 367-76.

Salo-Mullen, E.E., O'Reilly, E.M., Kelsen, D.P., et al. "Identification of germline genetic mutations in patients with pancreatic cancer." *Cancer* 121; no. 24 (2015): 4382-8.

Scurr, M.J., Brown, C.M., Costa Bento, D.F., et al. "Assessing the prognostic value of preoperative carcinoembryonic antigen-specific T-cell responses in colorectal cancer." *Journal of the National Cancer Institute* 107 (2015): djv001.

Sehdev, A., Gbolahan, O., Hancock, B.A., et al. "Germline and somatic DNA damage repair gene mutations and overall survival in metastatic pancreatic adenocarcinoma patients treated with FOLFIRINOX." *Clinical Cancer Research* 24, no. 24 (2018): 6204-11.

Seo, Y., Baba, H., Fukuda, T., et al. "High expression of vascular endothelial growth factor is associated with liver metastasis and a poor prognosis for patients with ductal pancreatic adenocarcinoma." *Cancer* 88, no. 10 (2000): 2239-45.

Sheanan, A.V., Biankin, A.V., Parish, C.R., et al. "Targeted therapies in the management of locally advanced and metastatic pancreatic cancer: a systematic review." *Oncotarget* 9, no. 30 (2018): 21613-27.

Shi, H., Li, J., Fu, D. "Process of hepatic metastasis from pancreatic cancer: biology with clinical significance." *Journal of Cancer Research & Clinical Oncology* 142, no. 6 (2016): 1137-61.

Shindo, K., Yu, J., Suenaga, M., et al. "Deleterious germline mutations in patients with apparently sporadic pancreatic adenocarcinoma." *Journal of Clinical Oncology* 35, no. 30 (2017): 3382-90.

Shroff, R.T., Hendifar, A., McWilliams, R.R., et al. "Rucaparib monotherapy in patients with pancreatic cancer and a known deleterious BRCA mutation." *JCO Precision Oncology* (2018) doi: 10.1200/PO.17.00316 [Epub 2018 May 16]

Siegel, R.L., Miller, K.D., Jemal, A. "Cancer Statistics, 2016." *CA: A Cancer Journal for Clinicians* 66, no.1 (2016): 7-30.

Singh, R.R., Goldberg, J., Varghese, A.M., et al. "Genomic profiling in pancreatic ductal adenocarcinoma and a pathway towards therapy individualization: a scoping review." *Cancer Treatment Reviews* 75, no. 5 (2019): 27-38.

Singhi, A.D., Ali, S.M., Lacy, J., et al. "Identification of targetable ALK rearrangements in pancreatic ductal adenocarcinoma." *Journal of the National Comprehensive Cancer Network* 15, no. 5 (2017): 555-62.

Singhi, A.D., Ishida, H., Ali, S.Z., et al. "A histomorphologic comparison of familial and sporadic pancreatic cancers." *Pancreatology* 15, no. 4 (2015): 387-91.

Slack, J.M. "Developmental biology of the pancreas." *Development* 121, no. 6 (1995): 1569-80.

Slavin, T., Neuhausen, S.L., Nehoray, B., et al. "The spectrum of genetic variants in hereditary pancreatic cancer includes Fanconi anemia genes." *Familial Cancer* 17, no. 2 (2018): 235-45.

Sohn, T.A., Yeo, C.J., Cameron, J.L., et al. "Resected adenocarcinoma of the pancreas – 616 patients: results, outcomes, and prognostic indicators" *Journal of Gastrointestinal Surgery* 4, no. 6 (2000): 567-79.

Steele, C.W., Karim, S.A., Leach, J.D.G., et al. "CXCR2 inhibition profoundly suppresses metastases and augments immunotherapy in pancreatic ductal adenocarcinoma." *Cancer Cell* 29, no. 6 (2016): 832-45.

Steinberg, W.M., Barkin, J.S., Bradley, E.L., et al. "Should patients with a strong family history of pancreatic cancer be screened on a periodic basis for cancer of the pancreas?" *Pancreas* 38, no. 5 (2009): e137- 50.

Stocken, D.D., Hassan, A.B., Altman, D.G., et al. "Modelling prognostic factors in advanced pancreatic cancer." *British Journal of Cancer* 99, no. (2008): 883-93.

Suzuki, R., Takagi, T., Hikichi, T., et al. "Derived neutrophil/lymphocyte ratio predicts gemcitabine therapy outcome in unresectable pancreatic cancer." *Oncology Letters* 11, no. 5 (2016): 3441-5.

Swords, D., Mulvihill, S.J., Firpo, M.A., et al. "Causes of death and conditional survival estimates of medium- and long-term survivors of pancreatic adenocarcinoma." *JAMA Oncology* 4, no. 8 (2018):1129-30.

Szkandera, J., Stotz, M., Absenger, G., et al. "Validation of C-reactive protein levels as a prognostic indicator for survival in a large cohort of pancreatic cancer patients." *British Journal of Cancer* 110, no. 1 (2014): 183-8.

Tabernero, J., Chiorean, E.G., Infante, J.R., et al. "Prognostic factors of survival in a randomized phase III trial (MPACT) of weekly nab-paclitaxel plus gemcitabine versus gemcitabine alone in patients with metastatic pancreatic cancer." *Oncologist* 20, no. 2 (2015): 143-50.

Takahashi, H., Morizane, C., Nomura, S., et al. "Phase II clinical trial of gemcitabine plus oxaliplatin combination therapy (GEMOX) in patients with advanced pancreatic adenocarcinoma with a family history of pancreatic/breast/ovarian/prostate cancer or personal history of breast/ovarian/prostate cancer (FABRIC study)." *Annals of Oncology* 29, Suppl 8 (2018): viii248-9.

Tanaka, T., Ikeda, M, Okusaka, T., et al. "Prognostic factors in japanese patients with advanced pancreatic cancer treated with single-agent gemcitabine as first-line therapy." *Japanese Journal of Clinical Oncology* 38, no. 11 (2008): 755-61.

Tas, F., Sen, F., Keskin, S., et al. "Prognostic factors in metastatic pancreatic cancer: older patients are associated with reduced overall survival." *Molecular and Clinical Oncology* 1, no. 4 (2013): 788-92.

Tas, F., Sen, F., Odabas, H., et al. "Performance status of patients is the major prognostic factor at all stages of pancreatic cancer." *International Journal of Clinical Oncology* 18, no. 5 (2013): 839-46.

ter Veer, E., van Rijssen, L.B., Besselink, M.G., et al. "Consensus statement on mandatory measurements in pancreatic cancer trials (COMM-PACT) for systemic treatment of unresectable disease." *Lancet Oncology* 19, no. 3 (2018): e151-60.

The Cancer Genome Atlas Research Network. "Integrated genomic characterization of pancreatic ductal adenocarcinoma." *Cancer Cell* 32, no. 2 (2017): 185-203.

Thomassen, I., Lemmens, V.E., Nienhuijs, S.W., et al. "Incidence, prognosis, and possible treatment strategies of peritoneal carcinomatosis of pancreatic origin: a population-based study." *Pancreas* 42, no. 1 (2013): 72-5.

Tsavaris, K., Kosmas, C., Papadoniou, N., et al. "CEA and CA 19-9 serum tumor markers as prognostic factors in patients with locally advanced (unresectable) or metastatic pancreatic adenocarcinoma: a retrospective analysis." *Journal of Chemotherapy* 21, no. 6 (2009): 673-80.

Van Cutsem, E., van de Velde, H., Karasek, P., et al. "Phase III trial of gemcitabine plus tipifarnib compared with gemcitabine plus placebo in advanced pancreatic cancer." *Journal of Clinical Oncology* 22, no.8 (2004): 1430-8.

Von Hoff, D.D., Ervin, T., Arena, F.P., et al. "Increased survival in pancreatic cancer with nab-paclitaxel plus gemcitabine." *New England Journal of Medicine* 369, no. 18 (2013): 1691-703.

Von Hoff, D.D., Ramanathan, R.K., Borad, M.J., et al. "Gemcitabine plus nab-paclitaxel is an active regimen in patients with advanced pancreatic cancer: a phase I/II trial." *Journal of Clinical Oncology* 29, no. 34 (2011): 4548-54.

Waddell, N., Pajic, M., Patch, A.-M., et al. "Whole genomes redefine the mutational landscape of pancreatic cancer." *Nature* 518, no. 7540 (2015): 495-501.

Wang, D.-S., Luo, H.-Y., Qiu, M.-Z., et al. "Comparison of the prognostic values of various inflammation based factors in patients with pancreatic cancer." *Medical Oncology* 29, no. 5 (2012): 3092-100.

Watanabe, I., Sasaki, S., Konishi, M., et al. "Onset symptoms and tumor locations as prognostic factors of pancreatic cancer." *Pancreas* 28, no. 2 (2004): 160-5.

Winograd, R., Byrne, K.T., Evans, R.A., et al. "Induction of T-cell immunity overcomes complete resistance to PD-1 and CTLA-4 blockade and improves survival in pancreatic carcinoma." *Cancer Immunology Research* 3, no. 4 (2015): 399-411.

Witkiewicz, A.K., McMillan, E.A., Balaji, U., et al. "Whole-exome sequencing of pancreatic cancer defines genetic diversity and therapeutic targets." *Nature Communications* 6 (2015): 6744.

Wu, L., Huang, P., Wang, F., et al. "Relationship between serum CA 19-9 and CEA levels and prognosis of pancreatic cancer." *Annals of Translational Medicine* 3, no. 21 (2015): 328.

Xue, P., Kanai, M., Mori, Y., et al. "Neutrophil-to-lymphocyte ratio for predicting palliative chemotherapy outcomes in advanced pancreatic cancer patients." *Cancer Medicine* 3, no. 2 (2014): 406-15.

Xue, P., Zhu, L., Wan, Z., et al. "A prognostic index model to predict the clinical outcomes for advanced pancreatic cancer patients following palliative chemotherapy." *Journal of Cancer Research and Clinical Oncology* 141, no. 9 (2015): 1653-60.

Yamada, S., Fujii T, Yabusaki N, et al. "Clinical implication of inflammation-based prognostic score in pancreatic cancer. Glasgow prognostic score is the most reliable parameter." *Medicine* 95, no. 18 (2016): e3582.

Yi, J.H., Lee, J., Park, S.H., et al. "A prognostic model to predict clinical outcomes with first-line gemcitabine-based chemotherapy in advanced pancreatic cancer." *Oncology* 80, no. 3-4 (2011): 175-80.

Yoo, T., Lee, W.J., Woo, S.M., et al. Pretreatment carbohydrate antigen 19-9 levels indicate tumor response, early distant metastasis, overall survival, and therapeutic selection in localized and unresectable pancreatic cancer. *International Journal of Radiation Oncology Biology Physics* 81, no. 4 (2011): e623-30.

Yu, S.-L., Xu, L.-T., Qi, Q., et al. "Serum lactate dehydrogenase predict prognosis and correlates with systemic inflammatory response in patients with advanced pancreatic cancer after gemcitabine-based chemotherapy." *Scientific Reports* 7 (2017): 45194.

Zhang, Y., Velez-Delgado, A., Mathew, E., et al. "Myeloid cells are required for PD-1/PD-L1 checkpoint activation and the establishment of an immunosuppressive environment in pancreatic cancer." *Gut* 66, no. 1 (2017): 124-36.

Zheng, B., Ohuchida, K., Yan, Z., et al. "Primary recurrence in the lung is related to favorable prognosis in patients with pancreatic cancer and postoperative recurrence." *World Journal of Surgery* 41, no. 11 (2017): 2858-66.

In: Horizons in Cancer Research. Volume 73 ISBN: 978-1-53616-273-8
Editor: Hiroto S. Watanabe

Chapter 2

NOVEL MOLECULAR MARKERS OF BREAST CANCER

K. Vaidyanathan*

Department of Molecular Biology, Amrita Institute of Medical Science & Research Center, Kochi, Kerala, India

ABSTRACT

Worldwide statistics suggest that breast cancer is the commonest cancer among women, accounting for nearly 25% of the total cancer cases. Though the survival rate is higher in the developed countries, it is poorer in the developing countries. Risk factors include advanced age, lack of childbearing and breastfeeding, Western dietary patterns and obesity, hormonal factors and genetic factors. Genetic factors include BRCA1 and BRCA2 gene mutations, and mutations/alterations in p53, PTEN, STK11, CHEK2, ATM, BRIK1 and PALB2 genes, and changes in DNA-repair genes like MSH2 and MLH1.

The advent of protein and DNA arrays and metabolomics platforms have led to accumulation of an immense amount of data, thereby providing crucial knowledge on the genetic signature of various types of breast

* Corresponding Author's E-mail: drkannanvaidyanathan@gmail.com.

cancer, and facilitating molecular diagnosis and therapy. Besides this, gene expression profiling and real-time PCR arrays are also used to explore cancer signaling pathways. Further, epigenetic markers have been discovered which are characteristic of certain breast cancer sub-types. . The challenge currently is to validate the utility of these markers. In future, Microarray-based and proteomic studies are expected to explore utilities and unearth new markers.

This chapter summarizes the current knowledge on the subject with an introduction on the "traditional" markers used in the diagnosis of breast cancer, followed by an account of the emerging markers

INTRODUCTION

Breast cancer is fast becoming one of the commonest causes of mortality and morbidity worldwide. There are many risk factors for the development of breast cancer. These include advanced age, lack of childbearing and breastfeeding, Western dietary patterns and obesity, hormonal factors and genetic factors. Genetic factors account for 10 - 15% of the cases, and they have distinctive phenotype. Mutations in BRCA1/BRCA2 genes are responsible for the majority of the cases, and they remain the most well-known. Mutations or alterations in p53, PTEN, STK11, CHEK2, ATM, BRIK1 and PALB2 genes, and DNA-repair genes like MSH2 and MLH1 are among the other well-known genetic changes.

Coming to the majority of breast cancers which are sporadic, there are a number of genes involved. One of the most aggressive genes which is linked to sporadic breast cancers is the gene, HER-2/neu. It has been identified that in the Western literature, about 25% of breast cancers are caused by over-expression of HER-2/neu gene. The relevance of this finding is that cancers which over-express HER-2/neu gene are highly resistant to conventional therapies and also highly aggressive in its biological characteristics, including local and distant metastasis (Vaidyanathan et al., 2010 and others). Mutations in HER-2/neu gene are not known to be a major factor in carcinogenesis; similarly, transcript levels are also not a major determinant, other than the secondary effect due to gene amplification.

Another major factor determining breast carcinogenesis is Hormone receptors; estrogen receptors and progesterone receptors, have been widely studied in the West, but large scale work has not yet been done in India (368 patients, Vaidyanathan et al., 2010 is the largest).

An equally important mechanism of carcinogenesis is epigenetic events. A number of studies done abroad have identified promoter hypermethylation and global hypomethylation as preliminary events in carcinogenesis. The second epigenetic event is related to histone acetylation levels.

Development of cancers in predisposed individuals requires environmental agents as well. External agents include radiation exposure, cigarette smoke and a Western lifestyle. Internal agents include estrogen, acquired mutations due to replication errors, and inherited mutations. These agents slowly lead to accumulation of genetic damage that eventually leads to tumors.

Amplification is a major mechanism of oncogenic activation in breast cancer. Oncogenes activated thus in breast cancer include EGFR, HER-2/neu, c-myc and cyclin D1, all of which are involved in cell division (Lin et al., 1984; Semba et al., 1985;Collins et al., 1982; Jiang et al., 1992; Devilee et al., 1994).

Loss of heterozygosity is responsible for development of tumors in predisposed individuals. It means loss of function of non-mutant normal allele; it can be either the primary or secondary event in carcinogenesis. Mutation of tumor suppressor genes is the commonest genetic alteration, andthe commonest gene is p53 (Hollstein et al., 1991), followed by p16/CDKN2/ARF and PTEN (Sherr 1996; Parsons 2004).

Somatic mutations can occur in both tumor suppressor genes and oncogenes. In tumor suppressor genes, both alleles must be inactivated during the development of tumors. For oncogenes, point mutations, amplifications, and translocations lead to activation. Distinct regulatory pathways, including those involved in cell cycle, apoptosis and genomic stability need to be compromised for tumor evolution. It is known that the clonal nature of tumors allows accumulation of multiple growth disruptions within the cell. Tumor development may take decades because multiple independent mutations must accumulate within a single clone. The rate of gene mutations is increased during clonal expansion of tumors; this phenomenon is referred to as genomic instability, which is a hallmark of most cancers (Hartwell & Kastan, 1994).

Pathways which normally repair are also disrupted in cancers.

Genomic integrity is normally maintained by the following systems:

1. Cell cycle system (CDK) (Spruck et al., 1999)
2. Repair pathways (Cleaver 1994; Syminngton, 2002; Petrini, 2000)
3. Checkpoint system (Elledge 1996)

Alterations in the checkpoint control pathways can occur due to ionizing radiations. These pathways basically regulate cell cycle and DNA repair systems. They enable the cell to repair itself before proceeding to the next cycle of division. The major pathway involves ATM, which transmits its signal to p53 to induce the cell to express p21 and arrest in G1 phase (Kastan et al., 1995). Repair after ionizing radiation is defective if p53 or ATM is non-functional. The cell can still undergo apoptosis if p53 is functional. However, if p53 is defective, the cell becomes polyploid (Fukasawa et al., 1996). Independent of p53, ATM may also phosphorylate CHK1/CHK2 pathways (checkpoint kinases) which induces inactivation mechanisms via CDC25 tyrosine phosphatases (Sorensen et al., 2003). A third branch of ATM pathway mediates repair of double-strand breaks via BRCA1 gene (Cortez et al., 1999). Genomic instability can be increased by a defect in cyclin D, p53, ATM and mismatch repair genes hMSH2 and hMLH1 (Elledge, 1996; Parsons et al., 1993).

Early-onset of Familial breast-ovarian cancer which affects women before the age of 50 is due to BRCA1 mutation while breast cancer without ovarian cancer is associated with BRCA or BRCA2 mutations. About 10% of women without a family history of breast cancer, but with a diagnosis of breast cancer before 35 years of age have a mutation in BRCA1.

The estrogen receptor is not reported to harbor mutations or loss of heterozygosity as with other genes. The loss of expression is rather due to hypermethylation of nearby CpG islands (Ottaviano et al., 1994).

Silencing of BRCA1 by promoter hypermethylation is reported in 10% of unselected breast cancers (Esteller et al., 2000). However, BRCA1 mutations are not reported in sporadic breast cancers (Futreal et al., 1994; Teng et al., 1996).

It is also seen that germ line mutations in E-cadherin gene predispose individuals to breast cancer. Loss of heterozygosity is another mechanism (chromosome 16q22.1 loss of heterozygosity, which contains CDH1 gene) that is the most frequent somatic genetic event in sporadic breast cancers. Poor E-cadherin expression is associated with tumor invasion and metastasis, correlating with metastasis and poor prognosis (Berx and Van Roy, 2001).

Cyclin D1 gene is amplified in 10% breast cancers and cyclin D1 protein in another 40% of cases (Dickson et al., 1995). Ras and HER-2/ neu signal exclusively through cyclin D1 (Yu et al., 2001). The role of cyclin D1 in tumrogenesis and promotion is currently in debate though it has key roles in differentiation as well (Lamb et al., 2003; Rowlands et al., 2004).

Inactivating mutations in p53 are found in about 60% of breast cancers. Germ line mutations are found in less than 1% of cancers, and are not accompanied by LOH (Gasco et al., 2002). The absence of functional p53 leads to genomic instability. Germ line and somatic mutations in PTEN are rare in the general population, but LOH occurs in 11 – 40% of sporadic breast cancers.

The role of hormones (estrogen) in breast carcinogenesis was recognized even in the 19th Century. As early as 1836, Cooper noted the relation of breast tumor growth with menstrual cycle. Beatson in 1896 reported regression of metastatic breast cancer with oopherectomy. About 70% of breast cancers express ER, and ER positive tumors proliferate in response to estrogen. Proliferation of ER positive cells occurs at the earliest stages of tumorigenesis. IGF-1, cyclin D1 and c-myc are transcriptional targets in the mitogenic response of breast to estrogen. Estrogen also activates MAPK pathway. However, ER positive tumors had better prognosis compared to ER negative ones. Estrogen receptor negative tumors had recurrences twice as much as those with tumors containing ER, independent of other prognostic markers. SERM including tamoxifen and raloxifen respond only in ER positive tumors (Andersen, 2002).

BRCA1 & BRCA2 Genes in Hereditary Breast Cancer

Genetic predisposition for early onset of familial breast cancer accounts for approximately 5 - 10% of all breast cancers, 7 - 10% of all ovarian cancers (Emery et al., 2001) and familial breast or breast and ovarian cancer (Miki et al., 1994; Wooster et al., 1995; Hall et al., 1990). Women who carry these BRCA1 or BRCA2 mutations have an estimated lifetime breast cancer risk between 60% and 85% and a lifetime ovarian cancer risk between 26% and 54% for BRCA1, and between 10% and 23% for BRCA2 (Brose et al., 2002; Easton et al., 1993; King et al., 2003; Antoniou et al., 2003).

The two main genes in hereditary breast cancer, viz., BRCA1 and BRCA2 have very large coding regions. BRCA1 has 27 coding exons and BRCA2 has 34 coding exons. In addition, mutations in the two genes can be spread throughout their coding region.

Although their mechanism of action is not yet fully elucidated, it is assumed that these genes play key roles in important cellular pathways, including response to DNA damage and transcription, and they interact with other proteins involved in DNA repair and apoptosis (Narod, 2004; Somasundaram et al., 2003). Genetic testing helps in identifying high risk individuals in families with inherited breast and/or ovarian cancer, and there are different management options available for mutation carriers.

Breast cancer is the most commonly occurring cancer among Indian women with relative proportion ranging from 19.3% to 27.5% (ICMR National Breast Cancer Registry, 2006). Significant variations in the relative contribution of mutations in BRCA1 and BRCA2 in the development of inherited familial breast and ovarian cancer and ovarian cancer have been reported (Liebens, 2007). However, the contribution of mutations in these two genes to breast cancer patients in the Indian familial breast or ovarian cancer remains relatively unexplored apart from a few small studies (Kumar et al., 2002; Saxena et al., 2002; Valarmathi et al., 2003, Valarmathi et al., 2004; Hedau et al., 2004; Rajkumar et al., 2003; Saxena et al., 2006, Mehta et al., 2018; Singh et al., 2018; Chakraborty et al., 2015).

More about BRCA1 and BRCA2

BRCA1 and BRCA2 are located on chromosomes 17q12-21 and 13q12-13, respectively (Couch et al., 2002). They encode multifunctional proteins, and contribute to homologous recombination, DNA damage response and regulation of transcription (Deng et al., 2006; Jasin, 2002; Mullan et al., 2006). They belong to a category of genes, known as caretaker genes, which maintain genomic integrity. Germline mutations in BRCA1/2 are responsible for 5% of breast cancers, and are inherited in an autosomal dominant manner (Wooster & Weber, 2003). Clinicopathological and histological character of BRCA1/2 mutation-carrying tumors are distinct and include early age of onset, high grade, ER/PR negativity, and high proliferation rate (Chappuis et al., 2000; Lakhani et al., 1998). Most commonly they are invasive ductal cancers, medullary sub-type and have prominent pushing margins and lymphocyte infiltration (Honrado et al., 2006; Philips, 2000). Tumors carrying BRCA2 mutation have rather less well-defined pathological characters. Even though they have higher grade, their ER/PR expression, pleomorphism, mitotic count and age distribution are similar to sporadic tumors (Lakhani et al., 2002).

Genomic instability includes aneuploidy, chromosomal and microsatellite instability, chromosomal aberrations, DNA amplifications, centrosome amplifications and micronuclei formation. In BRCA mutant tumors, genomic instability results from a failure of coordination of S-phase. (problems in these?)along with genomic instability are hallmarks of breast cancer (Kinzler & Vogelstein, 1997).

HER- 2/NEU GENE IN SPORADIC BREAST CANCER

HER-2/neu (c- Erb-B2) is a transmembrane growth factor receptor belonging to the type I receptor tyrosine kinase family of proteins. It is related to epidermal growth factor receptor (EGFR) and has high homology with other members of the EGFR family, which includes ErbB-1, ErbB-3 and ErbB-4 as well (Yamamoto et al., 1986; Bargman et al., 1986). The gene is located on chromosome 17q21 and encodes a 185 kDa protein (Fukushige tal, 1986). It has 1255 amino acids and is a highly phosphorylated protein. Normally ErbB-2 is expressed in a wide variety of tissues and is involved in normal growth, cell adhesion and development. HER-2/neu can both homodimerize and heterodimerize with other members of the EGFR family and activates a range of signal transduction pathways (Ullrich & Schlesinger, 1990; Woods et al., 2003).

HER-2/neu is an oncogene and is found to be overexpressed in 25 - 30% of sporadic breast cancers, according to international reports (Slamon et al., 1989; Di Fiorre et al., 1987, Slamon et al., 1987). However, Indian studies report a larger percentage of tumors as over-expressing HER-2/neu (Ray et al., 2004; Bhatavdekar et al., 2000) It is important to study whether HER-2/neu is overexpressed in breast cancer patients because these patients can opt for herceptin therapy, which is highly efficient for these patients (Slamon et al., 2001). Breast cancers which overexpress ErbB-2 are resistant to conventional therapy; they are also found to be more aggressive tumors compared to those which are negative (Slamon et al., 2001). It is also found that HER-2/neu positive tumors also frequently have tumors metastasis to lymph nodes (Allred et al., 1992, Gusterson et al., 1992). Estrogen (ER) and progesterone (PR) receptors are expressed in 70 - 80% and 60 - 70% cases of invasive ductal carcinoma respectively (Zafrani et al., 2000; Sastre- Garau et al., 1996). Patients with higher levels of HER-2/neu overexpression or amplification had statistically significantly lower levels of ER/PR than patients with lower levels of HER-2/neu overexpression or amplification. Because absolute HR levels are strongly related to response to hormone therapy in primary and advanced breast cancer, reduced ER/PR expression may be one mechanism to explain the relative resistance of HER-2/neu -

positive: Hormone receptor positive tumors to hormone therapy (Konecny et al., 2003). Mechanisms involved in HER-2/neu over expression include gene amplification and increased transcription, which in turn lead to increased protein turnover (Vernimmen et al., 2003). Gene amplification is known to be one of the major mechanisms responsible for HER-2/neu overexpression.

Literature generally reports an inverse correlation between HER-2 / neu gene and steroid receptors (estrogen receptor and progesterone receptor) (Zafrani et al., 2000; Satre Garau et al., 1996; Konecny et al., 2003). A positive correlation between lymph nodes and ErbB-2 overexpression has been reported (Querzoli et al., 1990; Tiwari et al., 1992). However, some studies found no association between lymph node status and ErbB-2 expression levels (Gullick et al., 1991). Even more overexpression of ErbB-2 is described in ductal carcinoma of the breast (Ariga et al., 2005). ErbB-2 overexpression either alone or along with other clinical parameters has been shown to be associated with poor prognosis in many studies (Marx et al., 1990; Guerin et al., 1988; Shackney et al., 2004; Nieto et al., 2004).

Other Cell-Cycle Associated Genes in Breast Cancer

Over-expression of C-MYC is reported in 5 - 50% of sporadic breast cancer in different studies. It is associated with poor prognosis similar to BRCA1-mutated cancers (Liao & Dickson, 2000). P53 mutations are seen in about half of patients carrying BRCA1/2 mutations. TP53 mutations are also seen in 1 in 5 sporadic breast cancers (Greenblatt et al., 2001). Higher frequency of E-cadherin mutations are seen in invasive lobular carcinoma. It is, however, less common in hereditary breast cancer (Arnes et al., 2005; Salahshor et al., 2001).

Loss of expression of p16 is seen in both familial and sporadic breast cancers (Esteller et al., 2001). p21 is associated with p53 and BRCA1 in breast cancer patients. It may have independent value as well (Osin &

Lakhani, 1999). Another cell cycle protein, p27, is associated with poor prognosis in breast cancer (Bloom & Pagano, 2003). The role of cyclin D1 in breast cancer is controversial and maybe only 1 in 10 breast cancers may harbour mutations in cyclin D1 (Armes et al., 1999). However, cyclin E is considered a marker for poor prognosis (Chappuis et al., 2005). Low expression of the apoptosis-associated gene, bcl-2, is characteristic of sporadic tumors (Osin & Lakhani, 1999).

Role of Promoter Hypermethylation in Breast Cancer

Both cancerous growth and metastasis involve coordinated silencing and activation of multiple genes. Programs of gene expression are controlled by the epigenome, including modification of histones (Strahl et al., 2000; Jenuwein et al., 2001), and the pattern of distribution of methyl residues at the 5' position of cytosine rings in the dinucleotide sequence CG (Razin et al., 1998; Razin et al., 1994). Active genes are associated with open hyperacetylated chromatin, which is hypomethylated at some residues such as K9 and K27 of the H3-histone tail and di- and tri-methylated at K4 (Strahl et al., 2000; Jenuwein et al., 2001). Regulatory regions of active genes associated with such chromatin structures are hypomethylated (Jenuwein et al., 2001).

Gene expression programs vary from cell type to cell type, and the epigenome is also unique for each cell type. Whereas the chromatin is associated with the genome, the methyl groups are part of its covalent chemical structure. Therefore, the pattern of methylation of DNA in a specific tissue is a stable mark of its identity and its unique gene expression program in contrast to chromatin, which is disrupted once the DNA is extracted and is hard to preserve in clinical samples. Profiling DNA methylation patterns provides therefore a stable image of the living genome. Primary and metastatic breast cancers display distinct methylation patterns (Huang et al., 1997; Huang et al., 1999; Chen et al., 2003).

The phenomenon of regional DNA hypermethylation and silencing of tumor suppressor genes in cancer has been the focus of attention in the last decade. A significant amount of data has established a list of genes hypermethylated in cancer, and whole genome approaches have identified methylation signatures of breast cancer cells (Huang et al., 1997; Huang et al., 1999; Chen et al., 2003). These methylation signatures, which are the unique combination of methylated CpG islands in a cancer cell can be correlated with breast cancer stage, and thus can be used as a diagnostic marker of breast cancer cells. In addition to their diagnostic value in breast cancer, it is clear from the repertoire of methylated genes that silencing of these genes by DNA methylation plays a role in the transformation process. Since it is well established that inhibitors of DNA methylation can induce tumor suppressor gene expression, it has also been proposed that DNA methylation inhibitors might serve as anticancer agents.

Amongst the methylated genes are tumor suppressor genes such as p16 whose methylation is proposed to silence this gene and override cell growth regulatory signals (Herman et al., 1995; Silva et al., 2003). p16 methylation in DNA prepared from plasma of breast cancer patients was associated with nodal metastasis (Hu et al., 2003). Hypermethylation of the promoter region of BRCA1 gene is reported to be an important event in sporadic breast cancers (Niwa et al., 2000; Rice et al., 2000) ?(Murata et al., 2002). Disruption of repair genes might increase sporadic mutations frequency, a hallmark of cancer cells. Steroid receptor genes family members such as the estrogen receptor (Piva et al., 1990) and retinoic acid beta 2 (RARβ2) receptor are methylated and silenced in a fraction of breast cancers (Sirchia et al., 2000; Widschwendter et al., 2000). Interaction of RARβ2 receptor with retinoic acid might have an antiproliferative effect, and its silencing confers a selective advantage on advanced breast cancer cells. Cell adhesion and cell surface molecules such as E-cadherin (Graff et al., 2000) and inhibitors of proteases such as TIMP-3 (Bachman et al., 1999), whose silencing promotes metastasis, are also found to be methylated in breast cancer.

Breast Cancer & Ionizing Radiation – Role of BRCA, ATM/ATR and Other Genes

Radiation has been indisputably proven to be a causative factor for the development of breast cancer. For instance, survivors of atomic bomb explosions in Japan have had a higher incidence of breast cancer (Land et al., 1995; Land et al., 2003). Also, breast cancer risk has been reported to be high in patients receiving diagnostic X-rays (Howe et al., 1996; Doody et al., 2000), and radiation treatment for benign conditions (Hildreth et al., 1989; Shore et al., 1986). It has also been observed that young women who received mantle radiation for Hodgkin's lymphoma also have increased risk of breast cancer (Travis et al., 2003, Bhatia et al., 1996; Wolden et al., 1998). Further, most studies show that dose-response relationship for breast cancer is almost linear (Preston et al., 2002). Considerable studies have shown that the effect of ionizing radiation on maturing breast lobules in adolescents enhances the risk of breast cancer (Tokunaga et al., 1994; Goss and Sierra, 1998). Exposures to ionizing radiation after the age of 50 years do not seem to increase the risk of breast cancer (Land et al., 2003).

The major mechanism by which ionizing radiation produces its effects is by a defect in DNA double strand break repair (DSB). A number of genes have been identified to be defective in cells exposed to ionizing radiation, including ATM/ATR, BRCA1 & BRCA2, p53 and Chk1 & Chk2 genes (Venkitaraman, 2001 Review).

BRCA1 mutant mice and cell lines are found to be hypersensitive to ionizing radiation (Gowen et al., 1998; Abbott et al., 1999). BRCA1 gene is also well known for its role in cell cycle regulation and DNA damage response (Reference). BRCA1 may be helped by other genes, especially BRCA2 and Rad51 in these functions (Chen et al., 1999).

ATM gene is mutated in some families with ataxia telangiectasia, features of which includes, among others, radiation sensitivity and an increased predisposition to cancer development. The effects produced by ATM defects are very similar to that produced by loss of BRCA1 (Venkitaraman, 2001 Review). AT carriers (AT mutation heterozygotes) may also have an increased predisposition to breast cancer (Swift et al., 1987; Swift et al., 1991; Vorechowsky et al., 1996; FitzGerald et al., 1997; Wooster et al., 1993; Athma et al., 1996; Easton et al., 1994; Cortessis et al., 1993). Studies in Scandinavian countries show that 9% of early-onset breast cancer patients have germline mutations in ATM gene (Schultz et al., 1999). This has, however, not been noticed in some other studies, probably reflecting a geographical variation (Chen et al., 1998). No study has been done in the Indian sub-continent in this area.

RECENT MARKERS IN BREAST CANCER

Recent evidence suggests that polymorphisms in genes involved in circadian rhythm, like *ARNTL*, *CLOCK*, *CRY1*, *CRY2*, *CSNK1E*, *NPAS2*, *NR1D1*, *NR1D2*, *PER1*, *PER2*, *PER3*, *RORA*, and *TIMELESS*, play a key role in the causation of many endocrine cancers, including breast cancer. These so-called circadian clock genes may promote tumor development and accelerate its fast progression. However, these studies need further validation (Morales-Santana et al., 2019).

New immunoglobulin genes, IGHA1, IGHD, IGHG1, IGHG3, IGLC2, and IGLJ3, and candidate genes, LST1 and IGHM have been implicated in TNBC. These genes were identified as tumor suppressor genes and are associated with relapse-free survival and distant metastasis-free survival, as per recent reports (Hsu et al., 2019).

The roles of GATA family members are being investigated and need further studies (Yu et al., 2019). Yu et al. opine that integrating genomic and transcriptomic profiles is very important and could greatly enhance the prognostic predictive efficiency in breast cancer. Their conclusion is based on a study of 810 breast cancer patients from the cancer-genome atlas (TCGA).

Ki-67 may help in the identification of intermediate prognostic groups with unfavourable prognosis and who may benefit from other therapy (Fasching et al., 2019). Studies continue to discover newer DNA methylation markers in breast cancer (de Almeida et al., 2019).

Many differentially expressed genes, which are grade-specific, including UBE2C and CCNB2 genes, the CDK1, KIF2C, NDC80, and CCNB2 genes, have been identified in breast cancer. Such genes collectively may function as good biomarkers for diagnosis and prognosis of breast cancer (Jayanthi et al., 2019).

The expression of Y-box binding protein, YBX1, is correlated with poor prognosis in breast cancer. YBX1 and its associated proteins are correlated negatively with ESR1 (Shibata et al.l, 2018).

Molecular profiling of circulating tumor cells (CTCs) reveals the role of various genes like CXCR4, uPAR, CD44, NANOG, which may be involved in cancer progression in early breast cancer (Markiewicz et al., 2019).

Mucin 1(MUC1) is a glycoprotein which predicts poor prognosis and is involved with metastasis and invasion? (Jing et al., 2019).

OCT4, SOX2, and NANOG positive expressions correlate with poor differentiation and advanced disease stage, and OCT4 and NANOG present with predictive values for poor overall survival in $HER2^{+}$breast cancer patients. These are transcription factors required for maintaining an embryonic pluripotent stem cell phenotype (Yang et al., 2018).

Differentially expressed genes, SFRP1, MMP7, CDH1, FAS, and UCP2 are potential biomarkers in breast cancer. Fusion genes, ESR1-C6orf97 with COBRA1-C9orf167 and VAPB-IKZF3 with ACACA-STAC2 were found in Luminal A and Luminal B breast cancer, respectively. However, these studies need further validation.

RET gene alterations, like amplification, missense mutations, known fusions, novel fusions, and rearrangements have been reported in breast cancer (Paratala et al., 2018).

KRAB-ZNF (Krüppel-associated box domain zinc finger) gene family consists of highly homologous genes, gene isoforms and pseudogenes. They act as epigenetic suppressors and may be potential tumor markers (Machnik et al., 2018). Differential expression of TFF1, TFF2 and TFF3 genes and proteins in breast cancer are described (Tolušić Levak et al., 2018).

Genome-wide DNA methylation studies on BRCA-like early breast cancer patients show altered methylation patterns in some genes; elevated methylation within the BRCA1 and SPHK2 promoter region and decreased methylation within the ADAP1, IGF2BP3 and SPATA13 promoter region were associated (Scott et al., 2018).

Paired box 5 (PAX5) methylation correlated with age, ER and PR status and might be a good biomarker for breast cancer (Li et al., 2018).

Recent evidence suggests the role of leptin and its signaling pathways in causing epithelial mesenchymal transition. Leptin is an adipokine, primarily associated with obesity. The association between breast cancer and obesity is well-known (Olea-Flores et al., 2018). There are other studies, however, which suggest that leptin and adiponectin are associated more with benign breast diseases than breast cancer (Quiroga-Morales et al., 2018).

Activin A, activin B, follistatin, follistatin-like (FSTL)-3, total IGF-1, total and intact insulin-like growth factor binding protein (IGFBP)-4 and pregnancy-associated plasma protein-A (PAPP-A) are ?associated with breast cancer (Panagiotou et al., 2019).

Forkhead Box M1 (FOXM1) is a key gene which performs multiple functions in TNBC. It may also function as an important therapeutic target in TNBC (Tan et al., 2019).

Early-grade cancer markers include GELS, DAPLE, HS90B, A1AT, IQCC, and CATD, as identified in a recent study based on 2D-DIGE (difference gel electrophoresis) (Pendharkar et al., 2018).

Osteopontin (OPN) is a predictive biomarker for breast cancer against anti-EGFR therapy (erlotinib). (Anborgh et al., 2018)

Recent studies indicate the role of ion channels in cancer pathogenesis. The expression of potassium ion channel gene, hERG1, is? associated with molecular sub-types in breast cancer, the highest expression is found in luminal A type whereas it is the lowest in basal-type cancers (Jorio et al., 2018).

CD24 is a glycosylated mucin-like antigen expressed on cell surface. In the recent years, CD24 has been identified as an oncogene and associated with metastasis promotion. CD24 is ?found to be elevated in breast cancer, compared to normal tissue (Jing et al., 2018).

Decreased expression of the breast cancer metastasis suppressor gene, BRMS1, is associated with poor prognosis and associated with clinic-pathological parameters in breast cancer (Lin et al., 2018).

Serum paraoxonase (PON) and arylesterase (ARE) levels decrease in breast cancer and this predicts neoadjuvant chemotherapy requirements (Okuturlar et al., 2018).

ALDH1, aldehyde dehydrogenase 1 gene, is associated with poor prognosis, high histological grade, ER/PR negativity and HER2 positivity in invasive breast cancer (Demir et al., 2018).

Mutations in RECQL, a member of the RecQ DNA helicase family, is associated with worse survival in breast cancer (Xu et al., 2018).

Survivin is an apoptosis inhibitor protein and plays an important role in tumor angiogenesis and cancer progression. It increases the risk of cancer independent of demographic factors (Gunaldi et al., 2018).

PAX2 (paired box 2) is a transcription factor involved in cell proliferation and carcinogenesis. Its expression is associated with better survival in tamoxifen-treated breast cancer (Jahangiri et al., 2018).

Chitinase 3 like 1 protein (CHI3L1) is associated with angiogenesis in invasive breast cancer and is associated with cancer progression (Rusak et al., 2018).

CONCLUSION

Many factors are involved in the causation of breast cancer. Traditional markers are widely used for the diagnosis and prognostication of breast cancer. However, a huge amount of research is being carried out around the globe to identify novel biomarkers. This is made possible with the advent of modern technology. There is a need for identification of markers which shall help to prognosticate as well as to focus on changes occurring in the cancer cell as a result of therapeutic agents. Such research is proceeding at a rapid pace. However, many of the novel molecular markers described in this text require proper validation and repetitive results in large-scale studies. The attempt of this chapter has been to summarize the most promising of these markers, after initially giving an insight on the more traditional markers. It should also be borne in mind that it is not possible to bring to light all such biomarkers in a single chapter. However, the more important ones have been highlighted. Future years shall determine the utility of some of these markers. Researchers may attempt to take up some of the interesting markers for their studies.

REFERENCES

Abbott, D. W., Thompson, M. E., Robinson-Benion, C., Tomlinson, G., Jensen, R. A. & Holt, J. T. (1999). BRCA1 expression restores radiation resistance in BRCA1- defective cancer cells through enhancement of transcription-coupled DNA repair. *J Biol Chem.*, *274*, 18808–12.

Allred, D. C., Clark, G. M., Tandon, A. K., Molina, R., Tormey, D. C., Osborne, C. K., et al. (1992). HER-2/neu in node- negative breast cancer: prognostic significance of over expression influenced by the presence of in situ carcinoma. *J Clin Oncol.*, *10*, 599-605.

Ames, B. N. & Gold, L. S. (1990). Too many rodent carcinogens: Mitogenesis increases mutagenesis. *Science.*, *249*, 970 – 971.

Anborgh, P. H., Lee, D. J., Stam, P. F., Tuck, A. B. & Chambers, A. F. (2018). Role of osteopontin as a predictive biomarker for anti-EGFR therapy in triple-negative breast cancer._*Expert Opin Ther Targets.*, *22*(8), 727-734. doi: 10.1080/14728222.2018.1502272. Epub 2018 Jul 26.

Andersen, E. (2002). The role of estrogen and progesterone receptors in human mammary development and tumorigenesis. *Breast Cancer Res.*, *4*, 197 – 201.

Antoniou, A., Pharoah, P. D., Narod, S., Risch, H. A., Eyfjord, J. E. & Hopper, J. L. (2003). Average risks of breast and ovarian cancer associated with BRCA1 or BRCA2 mutations detected in case Series unselected for family history: a combined analysis of 22 studies. *Am J Hum Genet.*, *72*, 1117-30.

Ariga, R., Zarif, A., Korasick, J., Reddy, V., Siziopikou, K. & Gattuso, P. (2005). Correlation of her-2/neu gene amplification with other prognostic and predictive factors in female breast carcinoma. *Breast J.*, *11*, 278-80.

Armes, J. E., Trute, L., White, D., et al. (1999). Distinct molecular pathogeneses of early-onset breast cancers in BRCA1 and BRCA2 mutation carriers: a population-based study. *Cancer Res.*, *59*(8), 2011–2017.

Arnes, J. B., Brunet, J. S., Stefansson, I., et al. (2005). Placental cadherin and the basal epithelial phenotype of BRCA1-related breast cancer. *Clin Cancer Res.*, *11*(11), 4003–4011.

Athma, P., Rappaport, R. & Swift, M. (1996). Molecular genotyping shows that ataxiatelangiectasia heterozygotes are predisposed to breast cancer. *Cancer Genet Cytogenet.*, *92*, 130–4.

Bachman, K. E., Herman, J. G., Corn, P. G., Merlo, A., Costello, J. F., Cavenee, W. K., et al. (1999). Methylation-associated silencing of the tissue inhibitor of metalloproteinase-3 gene suggest a suppressor role in kidney, brain, and other human cancers. *Cancer Res.*, *59*(4), 798–802.

Bargmann, C. I., Hung, M. C. & Wienberg, R. A. (1986). The neu oncogene encodes an epidermal growth factor receptor related protein. *Nature.*, *319*, 226-30.

Berx, G. & Van Roy, F. (2001). The E-cadherin/catenin complex: An important gatekeeper in breast cancer tumorigenensis and malignant progression. Breast *Cancer Res.*, *3*, 289 – 93.

Bhatavdekar, J. M., Patel, D. D., Shah, N. G., Vora, H. H., Suthar, T. P., Chikhlikar, P. R. et al.. (2000). Prognostic Significance of Immunohistochemically Localized Biomarkers in Stage II and Stage III Breast Cancer: A Multivariate Analysis. *Ann Surg Oncol.*, *7*, 305-311.

Bhatia, S., Robison, L. L., Oberlin, O., Greenberg, M., Bunin, G., Fossati-Bellani, F., et al.. (1996). Breast cancer and other second neoplasms after childhood Hodgkin's disease. *N Engl J Med.*, *334*, 745–51.

Bloom, J. & Pagano, M. (2003). Deregulated degradation of the cdk inhibitor p27 and malignant transformation. *Semin Cancer Biol.*, *13*(1), 41–47.

Brose, M. S., Rebbeck, T. R., Calzone, K. A., Stopfer, J. E., Nathanson, K. L. & Weber, B. L. (2002). Cancer risk estimates for BRCA1 mutation carriers identified in a risk evaluation program. *J Natl Cancer Inst.*, *94*, 1365-72.

Butterworth, B. & Slaga, T. (1991). Chemically-induced cell proliferation: Implications for risk assessment. New York, Wiley-Liss,

Chen, C. F., Chen, P. L., Zhong, Q., Sharp, Z. D. & Lee, W. H. (1999). Expression of BRC repeats in breast cancer cells disrupts the BRCA2–Rad51 complex and leads to radiation hypersensitivity and loss of G(2)/M checkpoint control, *J. Biol. Chem.*, *274*, 32931–32935.

Chakraborty, A., Banerjee, D., Basak, J. & Mukhopadhyay, A. (2015). Absence of 185delAG and 6174delT Mutations among Breast Cancer Patients of Eastern India. *Asian Pac J Cancer Prev.*, *6*(17), 7929-33.

Chappuis, P. O., Donato, E., Goffin, J. R., et al. (2005). Cyclin E expression in breast cancer: predicting germline BRCA1 mutations, prognosis and response to treatment. *Ann Oncol.*, *16*(5), 735–742.

Chappuis, P. O., Nethercot, V. & Foulkes, W. D. (2000). Clinico-pathological characteristics of BRCA1- and BRCA2-related breast cancer. *Semin Surg Oncol.*, *18*(4), 287–295.

Chen, C. M., Chen, H. L., Hsiau, T. H., Hsiau, A. H., Shi, H., Brock, G. J., et al.. (2003). Methylation target array for rapid analysis of CpG island hypermethylation in multiple tissue genomes. *Am J Pathol.*, *163*(1), 37–45.

Chen, J., Birkholtz, G. G., Lindblom, P., Rubio, C. & Lindblom, A. (1998). The role of ataxia-telangiectasia heterozygotes in familial breast cancer. *Cancer Res.*, *58*, 1376–9.

Cleaver, J. E. (1994). It was a very good year for DNA repair. *Cell.*, *76*, 1 – 4.

Cohen, S. M. & Ellwein, L. (1990). Cell proliferation in carcinogenesis. *Science.*, *249*, 1007 – 1011.

Collins, S. & Groudine, M. (1982). Amplification of endogenous myc related DNA sequences in a human myeloid leukemia cell line. *Nature.*, *298*, 679 – 81.

Cortessis, V., Ingles, S., Millikan, R., Diep, A., Gatti, R. A., Richardson, L., et al. (1993). Linkage analysis of DRD2, a marker linked to the ataxia-telangiectasia gene, in 64 families with premenopausal bilateral breast cancer. *Cancer Res.*, *53*, 5083–6.

Cortez, D., Wang, Y., Qin, J. & Elledge, S. J. (1999). Requirement of ATM-dependent phosphorylation of brca1 in the DNA damage response to double-strand breaks. *Science.*, *286* (5442), 1162 – 1166.

Couch, F. J. & Weber, B. L. (2002). Breast Cancer. In: *The genetic basis of human cancer.* (Vogelstein B, Kinzler KW, eds.) McGraw Hill, New York, NY. 549–581.

de Almeida, B. P., Apolónio, J. D., Binnie, A. & Castelo-Branco, P. (2019). Roadmap of DNA methylation in breast cancer identifies novel prognostic biomarkers. *BMC Cancer.*, *19*(1), 219. doi: 10.1186/s12885-019-5403-0.

Demir, H., Dulgar, O., Gulle, B. T., Turna, H. & Ilvan, S. (2018). Prognostic value of aldehyde dehydrogenase 1 (ALDH1) in invasive breast carcinomas. *Bosn J Basic Med Sci.*, *18*(4), 313-319. doi: 10.17305/bjbms.2018. 3094.

Deng, C. X. (2006). BRCA1: Cell cycle checkpoint, genetic instability, DNA damage response and cancer evolution. *Nucl Acids Res.*, *34*(5), 1416–1426.

Devilee, P., Schuuring, E., van de Vijver, M. J., et al. (1994). Recent developments in the molecular genetic understanding of breast cancer. *Crit Rev Oncogenesis.*, *5*, 247 – 70.

Di Fiore, P. P., Pierce, J. H., Kraus, M. H., Segatto, O., King, C. R. & Aaronson, S. A. (1987). erbB-2 is a potent oncogene when overexpressed in NIH/3T3 cells. *Science.*, *237*, 178- 82.

Dickson, C., Fantl, V., Gillett, C., et al. (1995). Amplification of chromosome band 11q13 and a role for cyclin D1 in human breast cancer. *Cancer Lett.*, *90*, 43 – 50.

Doody, M. M., Lonstein, J. E., Stovall, M., et al. (2000). Breast cancer mortality after diagnostic radiography: Findings from the US scoliosis cohort study. *Spine.*, *25*, 2052 – 63.

Easton, D. F., Bishop, D. T., Ford, D. & Crockford, G. P. (1993). Genetic linkage analysis in familial breast and ovarian cancer: results from 214 families. The Breast Cancer Linkage Consortium. *Am J Hum Genet.*, *52*, 678-701.

Easton, D. F. (1994). Cancer risks in A-T heterozygotes. *Int J Radiat Biol.*, 66(6 Suppl), S177–82.

Elledge, S. J. (1996). Cell cycle checkpoints: Preventing an identity crisis. *Science.*, *274*, 1664 – 71.

Emery, J., Lucassen, A. & Murphy, M. (2001). Common hereditary cancers and implications for primary care. *Lancet.*, *358*, 56-63

Esteller, M., Corn, P. G., Baylin, S. B. & Herman, J. G. (2001). A gene hypermethylation profile of human cancer. *Cancer Res.*, *61*(8), 3225–3229.

Esteller, M., Silva, J. M., Dominguez, G., et al. (2000). Promoter hypermethylation and BRCA1 inactivation in sporadic breast and ovarian tumors. *J Natl Cancer Inst.*, *92* (7), 564 – 569.

Fasching, P. A., Gass, P., Häberle, L., Volz, B., Hein, A., Hack, C. C., Lux, M. P., Jud, S. M., Hartmann, A., Beckmann, M. W., Slamon, D. J. & Erber, R. (2019). Prognostic effect of Ki-67 in common clinical subgroups of patients with HER2-negative, hormone receptor-positive early breast cancer. *Breast Cancer Res Treat.* doi: 10.1007/s10549-019-05198-9. [Epub ahead of print].

FitzGerald, M. G., Bean, J. M., Hegde, S. R., Unsal, H., MacDonald, D. J., Harkin, D. P., et al. (1997). Heterozygous ATM mutations do not contribute to early onset of breast cancer. *Nat Genet.*, *15*, 307–10.

Fukasawa, K., Choi, T., Kuriyama, R., et al. (1996). Abnormal centrosome amplification in the absence of p53. *Science.*, *271*, 1744 – 47.

Fukushige, S., Matsubara, K., Yoshida, M., Sasaki, M., Suzuki, T., Semba, K., et al. (1986). Localization of a novel v erbB related gene, c-erbB-2, on human chromosome 17 and its amplification in a gastric cancer cell line. *Mol Cell Biol.*, *6*, 955-8.

Futreal, P. A., Liu, Q., Shattuck-Eidens, D., et al. (1994). BRCA1 mutations in primary breast and ovarian carcinomas. *Science.*, *266*, 120 – 122.

Gasco, M., Shami, S. & Crook, T. (2002). The p53 pathway in breast cancer. *Breast Cancer Res.*, *4*, 70 – 76.

Goss, P. E. & Sierra, S. (1998). Current perspectives on radiation-induced breast cancer. *J Clin Oncol.*, *16*, 338–47.

Gowen, L. C., Avrutskaya, A. V., Latour, A. M., Koller, B. H. & Leadon, S. A. (1998). BRCA1 required for transcription-coupled repair of oxidative DNA damage. *Science.*, *281*, 1009–12.

Graff, J. R., Gabrielson, E., Fujii, H., Baylin, S. B. & Herman, J. G. (2000). Methylation patterns of the E-cadherin 50 CpG island are unstable and reflect the dynamic, heterogeneous loss of E-cadherin expression during metastatic progression. *J Biol Chem.*, *275*(4), 2727–32.

Greenblatt, M. S., Chappuis, P. O., Bond, J. P., Hamel, N. & Foulkes, W. D. (2001). TP53 mutations in breast cancer associated with BRCA1 or BRCA2 germ-line mutations: Distinctive spectrum and structural distribution. *Cancer Res.*, *61*(10), 4092–4097.

Guerin, M., Barrois, M., Terrier, M. J., Spielman, M. & Riou, G. (1988). Overexpression of either c-myc or c-erbB-2/neu proto-oncogenes in human breast carcinomas: correlation with poor prognosis. *Oncogene Res.*, *3*, 21-31.

Gullick, W. J., Love, S. B., Wright, C., Barnes, D. M., Gusterson, B., Harris, A. L., et al. (1991). C-erbB-2 protein overexpression in breast cancer is a risk factor in patients with involved and uninvolved lymph nodes. *Br J Cancer.*, *63*, 434-8.

Gunaldi, M., Isiksacan, N., Kocoglu, H., Okuturlar, Y., Gunaldi, O., Topcu, T. O. & Karabulut, M. (2018). The value of serum survivin level in early diagnosis of cancer. *J Cancer Res Ther.*, *14*(3), 570-573. doi: 10.4103/0973-1482.171369.

Gusterson, B. A., Gelber, R. D., Goldhirsch, A., Price, K. N., Save-Soderborgh, J., Anbazhagan, R., et al. (1992). Prognostic importance of c-erbB-2 expression in breast cancer International (Ludwig) Breast Cancer Study Group. *J Clin Oncol.*, *10*, 1049-56.

Hall, J. M., Lee, M. K., Newman, B., Morrow, J. E., Anderson, L. A., Huey, B., et al. (1990). Linkage of early-onset familial breast cancer to chromosome 17q21. *Science. 250*, 1684-9.

Hartwell, L. H. & Kastan, M. B. (1994). Cell cycle control and cancer. *Science.*, *266*, 1821 – 1828.

Hedau, S., Jain, N., Husain, S. A., Mandal, A. K., Ray, G., Shahid, M., et al. (2004). Novel germline mutations in breast cancer susceptibility genes

BRCA1, BRCA2 and p53 gene in breast cancer patients from India. *Breast Cancer Res Treat.*, *88*, 177-86.

Henderson, B., Ross, R. K., Pike, M., et al. (1982). Endogenous hormones as a major factor in human cancer. *Cancer Res.*, *42* (8), 3232 – 3239.

Herman, J. G., Merlo, A., Mao, L., Lapidus, R. G., Issa, J. P. & Davidson, N. E., et al. (1995). Inactivation of the CDKN2/p16/MTS1 gene is frequently associated with aberrant DNA methylation in all common human cancers. *Cancer Res.*, *55*(20), 4525–30.

Hildreth, N., Shore, R. & Dvoretsky, P. (1989). Risk of breast cancer after irradiation of the thymus in infancy. *N Engl J Med.*, *321*, 1281 – 4.

Hollstein, M., Sidransky, D., Vogelstein, B. & Harris, C. C. (1991). p53 mutations in human cancers. *Science.*, *253*, 49 – 53.

Honrado, E., Benâitez, J. & Palacios, J. (2006). Histopathology of BRCA1- and BRCA2-associated breast cancer. *Crit Rev Oncol Hemat.*, *59*(1), 27–39.

Howe, G. & McLaughlin, J. (1996). Breast cancer mortality between 1950 and 1987 after exposure to fractionated moderate dose rate ionizing radiation in the Canadian fluoroscopy cohort study and a comparison with breast cancer mortality in the atomic bomb survivors study. *Radiat Res.*, *145*, 694-707.

Hsu, H. M., Chu, C. M., Chang, Y. J., Yu, J. C., Chen, C. T., Jian, C. E., Lee, C. Y., Chiang, Y. T., Chang, C. W. & Chang, Y. T. (2019). Six novel immunoglobulin genes as biomarkers for better prognosis in triple-negative breast cancer by gene co-expression network analysis. *Sci Rep.*, *9*(1), 4484. doi: 10.1038/s41598-019-40826-w.

Hu, X. C., Wong, I. H. & Chow, L. W. (2003). Tumor-derived aberrant methylation in plasma of invasive ductal breast cancer patients: clinical implications. *Oncol Rep.*, *10*(6), 1811–5.

Huang, T. H., Laux, D. E., Hamlin, B. C., Tran, P., Tran, H. & Lubahn, D. B. (1997). Identification of DNA methylation markers for human breast carcinomas using the methylation-sensitive restriction fingerprinting technique. *Cancer Res.*, *57*(6), 1030–4.

Huang, T. H., Perry, M. R. & Laux, D. E. (1999). Methylation profiling of CpG islands in human breast cancer cells. *Hum Mol Genet.*, *8*(3), 459–70.

Indian Council of Medical Research NCRP. (2006). Consolidated Report of Population Based Cancer Registries, 2001-2004,

Iorio, J., Meattini, I., Bianchi, S., Bernini, M., Maragna, V., Dominici, L., Casella, D., Vezzosi, V., Orzalesi, L., Nori, J., Livi, L., Arcangeli, A. & Lastraioli, E. (2018). hERG1 channel expression associates with molecular subtypes and prognosis in breast cancer._*Cancer Cell Int.* doi: 10.1186/s12935-018-0592-1. eCollection 2018.

Jahangiri, R., Mosaffa, F., Gharib, M., Emami Razavi, A. N., Abdirad, A. & Jamialahmadi, K. (2018). PAX2 expression is correlated with better survival in tamoxifen-treated breast carcinoma patients._*Tissue Cell. 52*, 135-142. doi: 10.1016/j.tice.2018.05.005. Epub 2018 May 9.

Jasin, M. (2002). Homologous repair of DNA damage and tumorigenesis: The BRCA connection. *Oncogene.*, *21*(58), 8981–8993.

Jayanthi, V. S. P. K. S. A., Das, A. B. & Saxena, U. (2019). Grade-specific diagnostic and prognostic biomarkers in breast cancer. *Genomics.* . pii: S0888-7543(18)30459-2. doi: 10.1016/j.ygeno.2019.03.001. [Epub ahead of print].

Jenuwein, T. & Allis, C. D. (2001). Translating the histone code. *Science.*, *293*(5532), 1074–80.

Jiang, W., Kahn, S. M., Tomita, N., et al. (1992). Amplification and expression of the human cyclin D gene in esophageal cancer. *Cancer Res.*, *52*, 2980 – 83.

Jing, X., Cui, X., Liang, H., Hao, C., Yang, Z., Li, X., Yang, X. & Han, C. (2018). CD24 is a Potential Biomarker for Prognosis in Human Breast Carcinoma.___*Cell Physiol Biochem.*, *48*(1), 111-119. doi: 10.1159/000491667. Epub 2018 Jul 12.

Jing, X., Liang, H., Hao, C., Yang, X. & Cui, X. (2019). Overexpression of MUC1 predicts poor prognosis in patients with breast cancer._*Oncol Rep.*,_*41*(2), 801-810. doi: 10.3892/or.2018.6887. Epub 2018 Nov 27.

Kastan, M. B., Canman, C. E., Leonard, C. J. (1995). P53, cell cycle control and apoptosis: Implications for cancer. *Cancer Metastas Rev.*, *14*, 3 – 15.

King, M. C., Marks, J. H. & Mandell, J. B. (2003). Breast and ovarian cancer risks due to inherited mutations in BRCA1 and BRCA2. *Science.*, *302*, 643-6.

Kinzler, K. W. & Vogelstein, B. (1997). Cancer-susceptibility genes. Gatekeepers and caretakers. *Nature.*, *386*(6627), 761–763.

Konecny, G., Pauletti, G., Pegram, M., Untch, M., Dandekar, S., Aguilar, Z., et al. (2003). Quantitative association between HER-2/neu and steroid hormone receptors in hormone receptor positive primary breast cancer. *J Natl Cancer Inst.*, *95*, 142-53.

Kumar, B. V., Lakhotia, S., Ankathil, R., Madhavan, J., Jayaprakash, P. G., Nair, M. K., et al. (2002). Germline BRCA1 mutation analysis in Indian breast/ovarian cancer families. *Cancer Biol Ther.*, *1*, 18-21.

Lakhani, S. R., Jacquemier, J., Sloane, J. P., et al. (1998). Multifactorial analysis of differences between sporadic breast cancers and cancers involving BRCA1 and BRCA2 mutations. *J Natl Cancer Inst.*, *90*(15), 1138–1145.

Lakhani, S. R., Van De Vijver, M. J., Jacquemier, J., et al. (2002). The pathology of familial breast cancer: Predictive value of immunohistochemical markers estrogen receptor, progesterone receptor, HER-2, and p53 in patients with mutations in BRCA1 and BRCA2. *J Clin Oncol.*, *20*(9), 2310–2318.

Lamb, J., Ramaswamy, S., Ford, H., et al. (2003). A mechanism of cyclin D1 action encoded in the patterns of gene expression in human cancer. *Cell.*, *114*. 323 – 334.

Land, C. E., Tokunaga, M., Koyama, K., et al. (2003). Incidence of female breast cancer among atom bomb survivors, Hiroshima and Nagasaki, 1950-1990. *Radiat Res.*, *160*, 707-13.

Land, C. E. (1995). Studies of cancer and radiation dose among atomic bomb survivors. The example of breast cancer. *JAMA.*, *274*, 402–7.

Li, X., Huang, J., Luo, X., Yang, D., Yin, X., Peng, W., Bi, C., Ren, G., & Xiang, T. (2018). Paired box 5 is a novel marker of breast cancers that is frequently downregulated by methylation. *Int J Biol Sci., 14*(12), 1686-1695. doi: 10.7150/ijbs.27599. eCollection 2018.

Liao, D. J. & Dickson, R. B. (2000). c-Myc in breast cancer. *Endocr Relat Cancer., 7*(3), 143–164.

Liebens, F. P., Carly, B., Pastijn, A. & Rozenberg, S. (2007). Management of BRCA1/2 associated breast cancer: a systematic qualitative review of the state of knowledge in 2006. *Eur J Cancer., 43*, 238-57.

Lin, C. R., Chen, W. S., Kruiger, W., et al.. (1984). Expression cloning of human EGR receptor complementary DNA: Gene amplification and three related messenger RNA products in A431 cells. *Science., 224*, 843 – 8.

Lin, L., Cai, M., Dai, Y., Zheng, Z., Jiang, F., Shi, L., Pan, Y. & Song, H. B. (2018). Breast cancer metastasis suppressor gene, breast cancer metastasis suppressor 1, may be associated with clinicopathological features of breast cancer. *J Cancer Res Ther.*, S368-S374. doi: 10.4103/0973-1482.172125.

Machnik, M., Cylwa, R., Kiełczewski, K., Biecek, P., Liloglou, T., Mackiewicz, A. & Oleksiewicz, U. (2018). The expression signature of cancer-associated KRAB-ZNF factors identified in TCGA pan-cancer transcriptomic data. *Mol Oncol.* doi: 10.1002/1878-0261.12407. [Epub ahead of print].

Markiewicz, A., Topa, J., Nagel, A., Skokowski, J., Seroczynska, B., Stokowy, T., Welnicka-Jaskiewicz, M. & Zaczek, A. J. (2019). Spectrum of Epithelial-Mesenchymal Transition Phenotypes in Circulating Tumour Cells from Early Breast Cancer Patients. *Cancers (Basel)., 11*(1). pii: E59. doi: 10.3390/cancers11010059.

Marx, D., Schauer, A., Reiche, C., May, A., Ummenhofer, L., Reles, A., et al. (1990). c-erbB-2 expression in correlation to other biological parameters of breast cancer. *J Cancer Res Clin Oncol., 116*, 15-20.

Mehta, A., Vasudevan, S., Sharma, S. K., Kumar, D., Panigrahi, M., Suryavanshi, M. & Gupta, G. (2018). Germline BRCA1 and BRCA2 deleterious mutations and variants of unknown clinical significance associated with breast/ovarian cancer: a report from North India.

Cancer Manag Res., *10*, 6505-6516. doi: 10.2147/CMAR.S186563. eCollection 2018.

Miki, Y., Swensen, J., Shattuck-Eidens, D., Futreal, P. A., Harshman, K., Tavtigian, S., et al. (1994). A strong candidate for the breast and ovarian cancer susceptibility gene BRCA1. *Science.*, *266*, 66-71.

Morales-Santana, S., Morell, S., Leon, J., Carazo-Gallego, A., Jimenez-Lopez, J. C. & Morell, M. (2019). An Overview of the Polymorphisms of Circadian Genes Associated With Endocrine Cancer. *Front Endocrinol (Lausanne).*, Feb 26, *10*, 104. doi: 10.3389/fendo.2019.00104. eCollection 2019.

Mullan, P. B., Quinn, J. E. & Harkin, D. P. (2006). The role of BRCA1 in transcriptional regulation and cell cycle control. *Oncogene.*, *25*(43), 5854–5863.

Murata, H., Khattar, N. H., Kang, Y., Gu, L. & Li, G. M. (2002). Genetic and epigenetic modification of mismatch repair genes hMSH2 and hMLH1 in sporadic breast cancer with microsatellite instability. *Oncogene.*, *21*(37), 5696–703.

Narod, S. A. & Foulkes, W. D. (2004). BRCA1 and BRCA2: 1994 and beyond. *Nat Rev Cancer.*, *4*, 665-76.

Nieto, Y., Nawaz, S., Shpall, E. J., Bearman, S. I., Murphy, J. & Jones, R. B. (2004). Long-term analysis and prospective validation of a prognostic model for patients with high-risk primary breast cancer receiving high-dose chemotherapy. *Clin Cancer Res.*, *10*, 2609-17.

Niwa, Y., Oyama, T. & Nakajima, T. (2000). BRCA1 expression status in relation to DNA methylation of the BRCA1 promoter region in sporadic breast cancers. *Jpn J Cancer Res.*, *91*(5), 519–26.

Okuturlar, Y., Gunaldi, M., Kocoglu, H., Hursitoglu, M., Gedikbasi, A., Acarer, D., Harmankaya, O. & Kumbasar, A. (2018). Serum paraoxonase and arylesterase can be useful markers to predict neoadjuvant chemotherapy requirement in patients with breast cancer. *J Cancer Res Ther.*, S362-S367. doi: 10.4103/0973-1482.235355.

Olea-Flores, M., Juárez-Cruz, J. C., Mendoza-Catalán, M. A., Padilla-Benavides, T. & Navarro-Tito, N. (2018). Signaling Pathways Induced by Leptin during Epithelial-Mesenchymal Transition in Breast Cancer. *Int J Mol Sci.*, *6*, 19(11). pii: E3493. doi: 10.3390/ijms19113493.

Osin, P. P. & Lakhani, S. R. (1999). The pathology of familial breast cancer: Immunohistochemistry and molecular analysis. *Breast Cancer Res.*, *1*(1), 36–40.

Ottaviano, Y. L., Issa, J. P., Parl, F. F., et al. (1994). Methylation of the estrogen receptor gene CpG island marks loss of estrogen receptor expression in human breast cancer cells. *Cancer Res.*, 54, 2552 – 2555.

Panagiotou, G., Papakonstantinou, E., Vagionas, A., Polyzos, S. A. & Mantzoros, C. S. (2019). Serum Levels of Activins, Follistatins, and Growth Factors in Neoplasms of the Breast: A Case-Control Study. *J Clin Endocrinol Metab.*, *104*(2), 349-358. doi: 10.1210/jc.2018-01581.

Paratala, B. S., Chung, J. H., Williams, C. B., Yilmazel, B., Petrosky, W., Williams, K., Schrock, A. B., Gay, L. M., Lee, E., Dolfi, S. C., Pham, K., Lin, S., Yao, M., Kulkarni, A., DiClemente, F., Liu, C., Rodriguez-Rodriguez, L., Ganesan, S., Ross, J. S., Ali, S. M., Leyland-Jones, B. & Hirshfield, K. M. (2018). RET rearrangements are actionable alterations in breast cancer. *Nat Commun.*, *9*(1), 4821. doi: 10.1038/s41467-018-07341-4.

Parsons, R., Li, G. M., Longley, M. J., et al. (1993). Hypermutability and mismatch repair in RER+ tumor cells. *Cell.*, *75*, 1227 – 36.

Parsons, R. (2004). Human cancer, PTEN and PI-3-kinase pathway. *Semin Cell Div Biol.*, *15* (2), 171 – 76.

Pendharkar, N., Dhali, S. & Abhang, S. (2018). A Novel Strategy to Investigate Tissue-Secreted Tumor Microenvironmental Proteins in Serum toward Development of Breast Cancer Early Diagnosis Biomarker Signature. *Proteomics Clin Appl.*, e1700119. doi: 10.1002/prca.201700119. [Epub ahead of print].

Petrini, J. H. (2000). The Mre11 complex and ATM: Collaborating to navigate S phase. *Curr Opin Cell Biol.*, *12*, 293 – 296.

Phillips, K. A. (2000). Immunophenotypic and pathologic differences between BRCA1 and BRCA2 hereditary breast cancers. *J Clin Oncol.*, *18*(21 Suppl),107S–112S.

Piva, R., Rimondi, A. P., Hanau, S., Maestri, I., Alvisi, A., Kumar, V. L., et al. (1990). Different methylation of oestrogen receptor DNA in human breast carcinomas with and without oestrogen receptor. *Br J Cancer.*, *61*(2), 270–5.

Preston, D. L., Mattsson, A., Holmberg, E., et al. (2002). Radiation effects of breast cancer risk. A pooled analysis of 8 cohorts. *Radiat Res.*, *158*, 220 – 35.

Preston-Martin, S., Pike, M. C., Ross, R. K., et al. (1990). Increased cell division as a cause of human cancer. *Cancer Res.*, *50*, 7415 – 7421.

Querzoli, P., Marchetti, E., Fabris, G., Marzola, A., Ferretti, S., Iacobelli, S., et al.. (1990). Immunohistochemical expression of c-erbB-2 in human breast cancer by monoclonal antibody: correlation with lymph node and ER status. *Tumori.*, *76*, 461-4.

Quiroga-Morales, L. A., Sat-Muñoz, D., Martínez-Herrera, B. E., Alcántara-Cadillo, R. R., Macías-López, G. G., García-Cobián, T. A., Bañuelos-Rizo, M. & Balderas-Peña, L. M. A. (2018). Obesity and adipocytokines in breast cancer and benign breast disease_*Rev Med Inst Mex Seguro Soc.*, *56*(3), 246-254.

Rajkumar, T., Soumittra, N., Nancy, N. K., Swaminathan. R., Sridevi, V. & Shanta, V. (2003). BRCA1, BRCA2 and CHEK2 (1100 del C) germline mutations in hereditary breast and ovarian cancer families in South India. *Asian Pac J Cancer Prev.*, *4*, 203-8.

Ray, A., Sharma, B. K., Kaur, S., Sharma, S. & Sharma, J. K. (2004). Overexpression of c-erbB-2 oncoprotein and associated pathobiological factors in invasive primary breast cancer. *Indian J Exp Biol.*, *42*(3), 253-8.

Razin, A. & Szyf, M. (1984). DNA methylation patterns. Formation and function. *Biochim Biophys Acta.*, *782*(4), 331–42.

Razin, A. (1998). CpG methylation, chromatin structure and gene silencing-a three-way connection. *EMBO J.*, *17*(17), 4905–8.

Rice, J. C., Ozcelik, H., Maxeiner, P., Andrulis, I. & Futscher, B. W. (2000). Methylation of the BRCA1 promoter is associated with decreased BRCA1 mRNA levels in clinical breast cancer specimens. *Carcinogenesis.*, *21*(9), 1761–5.

Rowlands, T. M., Pechenkina, I. V., Hatsell, S., et al. (2004). Beta catenin and cyclin D1: Connecting development to breast cancer. *Cell cycle.*, *3*, 145 – 148.

Rusak, A., Jablonska, K., Piotrowska, A., Grzegrzolka, J., Nowak, A., Wojnar, A. & Dziegiel, P. (2018). The Role of CHI3L1 Expression in Angiogenesis in Invasive Ductal Breast Carcinoma. *Anticancer Res.*, *38*(6), 3357-3366. doi: 10.21873/anticanres.12602.

Salahshor, S., Haixin, L., Huo, H., et al. (2001). Low frequency of Ecadherin alterations in familial breast cancer. *Breast Cancer Res.*, *3*(3), 199–207.

Sastre-Garau, X., Jouve, M., Asselain, B., Vincent – Salomon, A., Beuzboc, P., Dorval, T., et al. (1996). Infiltrating lobular carcinoma of the breast; clinico-pathologic analysis of 975 cases with reference to data on conservative therapy and metastatic patterns. *Cancer.*, *77*, 113-120.

Saxena, S., Chakraborty, A., Kaushal, M., Kotwal, S., Bhatanager, D. & Mohil, R. S. (2006). Contribution of germline BRCA1 and BRCA2 sequence alterations to breast cancer in Northern India. *BMC Med Genet.*, *7*, 75.

Saxena, S., Szabo, C. I., Chopin, S., Barjhoux, L., Sinilnikova, O., Lenoir, G., et al. (2002). BRCA1 and BRCA2 in Indian breast cancer patients. *Hum Mutat.*, *20*, 473-4.

Schultz, L. B. & Weber, B. L. (1999). Recent advances in breast cancer biology. *Curr Opin Oncol.*, *11*, 429–34.

Scott, C. M., Wong, E. M., Joo, J. E., Dugué, P. A., Jung, C. H., O'Callaghan, N., Dowty, J., Giles, G. G., Hopper, J. L. & Southey, M. C. (2018). Genome-wide DNA methylation assessment of 'BRCA1-like' early-onset breast cancer: Data from the Australian Breast Cancer Family Registry. *Exp Mol Pathol.*, *105*(3), 404-410. doi: 10.1016/j.yexmp.2018.11.006. Epub 2018 Nov 10.

Semba, K., Kamata, N., Toyoshima, K., et al.. (1985). A v-erbB-related protooncogene, c- erbB-2, is distinct from the c-erbB-1/epidermal growth factor gene and is amplified in a human salivary gland adenocarcinoma. *Proc Natl Acad Sci USA.*, *82*, 6497 – 501.

Shackney, S. E., Smith, C. A., Pollice, A., Brown, K., Day, R., Julian, T., et al. (2004). Intracellular patterns of Her-2/neu, ras and ploidy abnormalities in primary breast cancers predict postoperative clinical disease-free survival. *Clin Cancer Res.*, *10*, 3042-52.

Sherr, C. J. (1996). Cancer cell cycles. *Science.*, *274*, 1672 – 77.

Shibata, T., Tokunaga, E., Hattori, S., Watari, K., Murakami, Y., Yamashita, N., Oki, E., Itou, J., Toi, M., Maehara, Y., Kuwano, M. & Ono, M. (2018). Y-box binding protein YBX1 and its correlated genes as biomarkers for poor outcomes in patients with breast cancer. *Oncotarget.*, *9*(98), 37216-37228. doi: 10.18632/oncotarget.26469. eCollection 2018 Dec 14.

Shore, R. E., Hilreth, N., Woodard, E., et al. (1986). Breast cancer among women given X-ray therapy for acute post-partum mastitis. *J Natl Cancer Inst.*, *77*, 689 – 96.

Silva, J., Silva, J. M., Dominguez, G., Garcia, J. M., Cantos, B., Rodriguez, R., et al. (2003). Concomitant expression of p16INK4a and p14ARF in primary breast cancer and analysis of inactivation mechanisms. *J Pathol.*, *199*(3), 289–97.

Singh, J., Thota, N., Singh, S., Padhi, S., Mohan, P., Deshwal, S., Sur, S., Ghosh, M., Agarwal, A., Sarin, R., Ahmed, R., Almel, S., Chakraborti, B., Raina, V., DadiReddy, P. K., Smruti, B. K., Rajappa, S., Dodagoudar, C., Aggarwal, S., Singhal, M., Joshi, A., Kumar, R., Kumar, A., Mishra, D. K., Arora, N., Karaba, A., Sankaran, S., Katragadda, S., Ghosh, A., Veeramachaneni, V., Hariharan, R. & Mannan, A. U. (2018). Screening of over 1000 Indian patients with breast and/or ovarian cancer with a multi-gene panel: prevalence of BRCA1/2 and non-BRCA mutations. *Breast Cancer Res Treat.*, *170*(1), 189-196. doi: 10.1007/s10549-018-4726-x. Epub 2018 Feb 22.

Sirchia, S. M., Ferguson, A. T., Sironi, E., Subramanyan, S., Orlandi, R., Sukumar, S., et al. (2000). Evidence of epigenetic changes affecting the chromatin state of the retinoic acid receptor beta2 promoter in breast cancer cells. *Oncogene.*, *19*(12), 1556–63.

Slamon, D. J., Clark, G. M., Wong, S. G., Levin, W. J., Ullrich, A. & McGuire, W. L. (1987). Human breast cancer: Correlation of relapse and survival with amplification of the HER-2/neu oncogene. *Science.*, *235*, 177-82.

Slamon, D. J., Godolphin, W., Jones, L. A., Holt, J. A., Wong, S. G., Keith, D. E., et al. (1989). Studies of the HER-2/neu proto oncogene in human breast and ovarian cancer. *Science.*, *244*, 707-12.

Slamon, D. J., Leyland-Jones, B., Shak, S., Fuchs, H., Paton, V., Bajamonde, A., et al. (2001). Use of chemotherapy plus a monoclonal antibody against HER2 for metastatic breast cancer that overexpresses HER-2. *N Eng J Med.*, *344*, 783-92.

Somasundaram, K. (2003). Breast cancer gene 1 (BRCA1): role in cell cycle regulation and DNA repair--perhaps through transcription. *J Cell Biochem.*, *88*, 1084-91.

Sorensen, C. S., Syljuasen, R. G., Falck, J., et al. (2003). Chk1 regulates the S phase checkpoint by coupling the physiological turnover and ionizing radiation induced accelerated proteolysis of Cdc25A. *Cancer cell.*, *3*, 247 – 258.

Spruck, C. H., Won, K. A. & Reed, S. I. (1999). Deregulated cyclin E induces chromosomal instability. *Nature.*, *401*, 297 – 300.

Strahl, B. D. & Allis, C. D. (2000). The language of covalent histone modifications. *Nature.*, *403*(6765), 41–5.

Swift, M., Morrell, D., Massey, R. B. & Chase, C. L. (1991). Incidence of cancer in 161 families affected by ataxia-telangiectasia. *N Engl J Med.*, *325*, 1831–6.

Swift, M., Reitnauer, P. J., Morrell, D. & Chase, C. L. (1987). Breast and other cancers in families with ataxia-telangiectasia. *N Engl J Med.*, *316*, 1289–94.

Symington, L. S. (2002). Role of RAD52 epistasis group genes in homologous recombination and double strand break repair. *Microbiol Mol Biol Rev.*, *66* (4), 630 – 670.

Tan, Y., Wang, Q., Xie, Y., Qiao, X., Zhang, S., Wang, Y., Yang, Y. & Zhang, B. (2019). Identification of FOXM1 as a specific marker for triple-negative breast cancer. *Int J Oncol.* 54(1):87-97. doi: 10.3892/ijo.2018.4598. Epub 2018 Oct 19.

Teng, D., Bogden, R., Mitchell, J., et al. (1996). Low incidence of BRCA2 mutations in breast carcinoma and other cancers. *Nature Genetics.*, *13*, 241 – 244.

Tiwari, R. K., Borgen, P. I., Wong, G. Y., Cordon-Cardo, C. & Osborne, M. P. (1992). HER-2/neu amplification and overexpression in primary human breast cancer is associated with early metastasis. *Anticancer Res.*, *12*, 419-25.

Tokunaga, M., Land, C. E., Tokuoka, S., Nishimori, I., Soda, M. & Akiba, S. (1994). Incidence of female breast cancer among atomic bomb survivors, 1950–1985. *Radiat Res.*, *138*, 209–23.

Tolušić Levak, M., Mihalj, M., Koprivčić, I., Lovrić, I., Novak, S., Bijelić, N., Baus-Lončar, M., Belovari, T., Kralik, K. & Pauzar, B. (2018). Differential Expression of TFF Genes and Proteins in Breast Tumors. *Acta Clin Croat.*, *57*(2), 264-277. doi: 10.20471/acc.2018.57.02.06.

Travis, L. B., Hill, D. A., Dores, G. M., et al. (2003). Breast cancer following radiotherapy and chemotherapy among young women with Hodgkin's disease. *JAMA.*, *290*, 465 – 75.

Ullrich, A. & Schlesinger, J. (1990). Signal transduction by receptors with tyrosine kinase activity. *Cell.*, *61*, 203-212.

Vaidyanathan, K., Kumar, P., Reddy, C. O., Deshmane, V., Somasundaram, K. & Mukherjee, G. (2010). "ErbB-2 expression and its association with other biological parameters of breast cancer among Indian women" - *Ind J Cancer.*, *47* (1), 14 – 21.

Vaidyanathan, K., Lakhotia, S., Ravishankar, H. M., Tabassum, U., Mukherjee, G. & Somsundaram, K. (2009). BRCA1 and BRCA2 Germline Mutation Analysis among Indian Women: Identification of Four Novel Mutations and High Frequency Occurrence of 185delAG Mutation with Independent Origin. *Journal of Biosciences.*, *34*(3), 415–422.

Valarmathi, M. T. A. A., Deo, S. S., Shukla, N. K. & Das, S. N. (2003). BRCA1 germline mutations in Indian familial breast cancer. *Hum Mutat.*, *21*, 98-9.

Valarmathi, M. T., Sawhney, M., Deo, S. S., Shukla, N. K. & Das, S. N. (2004). Novel germline mutations in the BRCA1 and BRCA2 genes in Indian breast and breast-ovarian cancer families. *Hum Mutat.*, *23*, 205.

Venkitaraman, A. R. (2001). Functions of BRCA1 and BRCA2 in the biological response to DNA damage. *Journal of Cell Science., 114*, 3591-98.

Vernimmen, D., Gueders, M., Pisvin, S., Delvenne, P. & Winkler, R. (2003). Different mechanisms are implicated in ErbB-2 gene over expression in breast and in other cancers. *Br J Cancer., 89*, 899-906.

Vorechovsky, I., Luo, L., Lindblom, A., Negrini, M., Webster, A. D., Croce, C. M,, et al. (1996). ATM mutations in cancer families. *Cancer Res., 56*, 4130–3.

Wang, R., Li, J., Yin, C., Zhao, D. & Yin, L. (2018). Identification of differentially expressed genes and typical fusion genes associated with three subtypes of breast cancer._*Breast Cancer*. doi: 10.1007/s12282-018-0924-y. [Epub ahead of print].

Widschwendter, M., Berger, J., Hermann, M., Muller, H. M., Amberger, A., Zeschnigk, M., et al.. (2000). Methylation and silencing of the retinoic acid receptor-beta2 gene in breast cancer. *J Natl Cancer Inst., 92*(10), 826–32.

Wolden, S. L., Lamborn, K. R., Cleary, S. F., Tate, D. J. & Donaldson, S. S. (1998). Second cancers following pediatric Hodgkin's disease. *J Clin Oncol., 16*, 536–44.

Woods Ignatoski, K. M., Livant, D. L., Markwart, S., Grewal, N. K. & Ethier, S. P. (2003). The role of phosphatidylinositol 3' kinase and its downstream signals in erbB-2 mediated transformation. *Mol Cancer Res., 1*, 551- 60.

Wooster, R., Bignell, G., Lancaster, J., Swift, S., Seal, S., Mangion, J., et al. (1995). Identification of the breast cancer susceptibility gene BRCA2. *Nature., 378*, 789-92.

Wooster, R., Ford, D., Mangion, J., Ponder, B. A., Peto, J., Easton, D. F., et al. (1993). Absence of linkage to the ataxia telangiectasia locus in familial breast cancer. *Hum Genet., 92*, 91–4.

Wooster, R. & Weber, B. L. (2003). Breast and ovarian cancer. *New Engl J Med., 348*(23), 2339–2347.

Xu, H., Xu, Y., Ouyang, T., Li, J., Wang, T., Fan, Z., Fan, T., Lin, B. & Xie, Y. (2018). Low expression of RECQL is associated with poor prognosis in Chinese breast cancer patients._*BMC Cancer.*, *18*(1), 662. doi: 10.1186/s12885-018-4585-1.

Yamamoto, T., Ikawa, S., Akiyama, T., Semba, K., Nomura, N., Miyajima, N., et al. (1986). Similarity of protein encoded by the human c-erbB-2 gene to epidermal growth factor receptor. *Nature.*, *319*, 230-4.

Yang, F., Zhang, J. & Yang, H. (2018). OCT4, SOX2, and NANOG positive expression correlates with poor differentiation, advanced disease stages, and worse overall survival in $HER2^+$ breast cancer patients._*Onco Targets Ther.*, *11*, 7873-7881. doi: 10.2147/OTT.S173522. eCollection 2018.

Yu, C., Qin, N., Pu, Z., Song, C., Wang, C., Chen, J., Dai, J., Ma, H., Jiang, T. & Jiang, Y. (2019). Integrating of genomic and transcriptomic profiles for the prognostic assessment of breast cancer. *Breast Cancer Res Treat*. doi: 10.1007/s10549-019-05177-0. [Epub ahead of print].

Yu, Q., Geng, Y. & Sicinski, P. (2001). Specific protection against breast cancers by cyclin D1 ablation. *Nature.*, *411*, 1017 – 1021.

Yu, S., Jiang, X., Li, J., Li, C., Guo, M., Ye, F., Zhang, M., Jiao, Y. & Guo, B. (2019). Comprehensive analysis of the GATA transcription factor gene family in breast carcinoma using gene microarrays, online databases and integrated bioinformatics. *Sci Rep.*, *9*(1), 4467. doi: 10.1038/s41598-019-40811-3.

Zafrani, B., Aubriot, M. H., Mouret, E., De Crémoux, P., De Rycke, Y., Nicolas, A., et al. (2000). High sensitivity and specificity of immunohistochemistry for the detection of hormone receptors in breast carcinoma: comparison with biochemical determination in a prospective study of 793 cases *Histopathology.*, *37*, 536-45.

Biographical Sketch

Name: Kannan Vaidyanathan

Affiliation: Amrita Institute of Medical Sciences & Research Center, Kochi, Kerala, India

Education: MBBS, MD (Biochemistry)

Business Address: Professor & Head, Department of Molecular Biology, Amrita Institute of Medical Sciences & Research Center, Kochi, Kerala, India

Research and Professional Experience: 20 Years

Professional Appointments:

Lecturer, Dept of Biochemistry, Medical College, Kottayam - 1 yr and 3 months (Jul '99 – Aug'00, Aug '03 – Sept '03)

Assistant Professor, Co-operative Medical College, Dept of Biochemistry – 6 ½ months (01.02.06 – 16.08.06)

Clinical Assistant Professor, Dept of Biochemistry, Amrita Institute of Medical Sciences, AIMS Ponekkara PO, Kochi – 682 041 (17.08.06 – 23.12.09)

Clinical Associate Professor, Dept of Biochemistry, Amrita Institute of Medical Sciences, AIMS Ponekkara PO, Kochi – 682 041 (24.12.09 – 23.12.12)

Clinical Additional Professor, Dept of Biochemistry, Amrita School of Medicine, AIMS Ponekkara PO, Kochi – 682 041 (24.12.12 – 02.03.2013)

Professor & Head, Department of Biochemistry, Pushpagiri Institute of Medical Science, Tiruvalla 689 101 (04.03.2013 – 30.04.2017)

Deputy Medical Superintendent (Central Laboratory), Pushpagiri Medical College Hospital, Tiruvalla, Kerala (01.01.2014 – 30.09.2018)

In-Charge, Metabolic Disorders Laboratory at Amrita Institute of Medical Sciences, Kochi and Arterial blood gases (ABG) facility at Amrita Institute of Medical Sciences, Kochi (01.09.2006 – 02.03.2013)

Deputy Technical Manager, Amrita Laboratory Services, Amrita Institute of Medical Sciences, Kochi (01.04.2007 - 02.03.2013)

Coordinator, MSc Program, Amrita School of Medicine, Kochi (01.03.2012 – 02.03.2013)

Professor, Department of Biochemistry, Pushpagiri Institute of Medical Science and Research Center, Tiruvalla, Kerala, INDIA - 689 101 (04.03.2013 – 02.05.2019)

Scientist, Pushpagiri Research Center, Pushpagiri Institute of Medical Science and Research Center, Tiruvalla, Kerala, INDIA - 689 101 (01.05.2017 – 02.05.2019)

Honors:

Scholarships and fellowships:

1. Postdoctoral fellowship – Department of Biotechnology (DBT-PDF) Department of Microbiology & Cell Biology, Indian Institute of Science, Bangalore
2. APFCB (Asia Pacific Federation of Clinical Biochemists) International Silver Jubilee scholarship, November 2007. Travel fellowship for Singapore Dollars 2500 and free registration for APFCB Conference (worth USD 500) conference at Beijing China during November 2007. Presented a scientific article during the conference titled - "Role of BRCA1 and BRCA2 genes in hereditary breast/ovarian cancer". Authors - Kannan Vaidyanathan, HM Ravi Shanker, Smita Lakhotia, Kumaravel Somasundaram & Geeta Mukherjee

Awards won:

"KP Sinha – PS Krishnan Award" - Best Paper award for best original research paper published in Indian Journal of Clinical Biochemistry published for the year 2011. For the paper . "Diagnosis of organic acidurias: methylmalonic aciduria, propionic aciduria, isovaleric aciduria and maple syrup urine disease in children: Two years' experience at a tertiary care centre". Indian Journal of Clinical Biochemistry (Oct – Dec 2011), 26 (4):

347 – 353 – Authors - MP Narayanan, K Vaidyanathan, KP Vinayan, DM Vasudevan.

Other special achievements:

1. Examiner for MBBS (Biochemistry), BDS, PhD, and MSc (Medical Biochemistry & Allied Health Sciences)
2. Joint Organizing Secretary, ACBICON 2009, Annual National Conference of Association of Clinical Biochemists of India, 5th – 7th November, 2009.
3. Kerala State Representative of Association of Clinical Biochemists of India (ACBI) – 2008 – 2009.
4. Executive Member, Association of Clinical Biochemists of India (ACBI) - 2010 onwards.
5. Secretary, Indian Board of Clinical Biochemistry (IBMB) – December 2012 onwards
6. Approved PhD guide of Kerala University of Health Sciences – Medicine – 2016 onwards.
7. South Zone representative, Association of Clinical Biochemists of India (ACBI) - 2016 onwards.
8. Institutional Ethics Committee Member, Pushpagiri Institute of Medical Science & Research Center, Tiruvalla, Kerala and Believers Church Medical College Hospital, Tiruvalla, Kerala.
9. Clinical Laboratory experience for over 16 years, more than 10 years in ISO 15189 for medical laboratories, certified internal assessor.
10. Managing Editor, Indian Journal of Clinical Biochemistry (IJCB) Indexed in PubMed Central and published by Springer.
11. International Lead Assessor, as per ISO 15189:2012.

Publications from the Last 3 Years:

Textbooks:

[1] Vasudevan, DM; Sreekumari, S; Vaidyanathan, K. "Textbook of Biochemistry (For Medical Students)" Published by Jaypee Brothers

(Now in 8th Ed, 2016) ISBN: 978-93-5090-530-2. This textbook is available in Spanish language and is published by Jaypee Highlights in Spanish. This textbook is also available in Slovenian. http://www.jaypeebrothers.com/pgDetails.aspx?book_id=978938599 9741.

[2] Vasudevan, DM; Sreekumari, S; Vaidyanathan, K. "Textbook of Biochemistry for Dental students Published by Jaypee Brothers. ISBN: 978-93-5025-488-2 (3rd Ed, 2017)

[3] Vaidyanathan, K. "NMR spectroscopy in medical diagnosis – Recent Developments" Chapter in the book series "NMR spectroscopy in Medical Diagnosis, Food Sciences, and Molecular Identification in Structural Biology/Secondary Metabolites; Applications of NMR Spectroscopy" Editors Prof. Atta-ur-Rahman, M Iqbal Chaudhary. Bantham Science Publishers.

Journal Articles

[1] Gaddam, V. L., Gowda, V. & Vaidyanathan, K. (2016). Comparison of the effectiveness of horizontal integration with traditional teaching approach in first-year MBBS students. International *Journal of Medical Science and Public Health.*, *5* (07) (Online First).

[2] Vijayakumar, M., Vasudevan, D. M., Sundaram, K. R., Krishnan, S., Vaidyanathan, K., Nandakumar, S., Chandrasekhar, R. & Mathew, N. (2016). A randomized study of coconut oil versus sunflower oil on cardiovascular risk factors in patients with stable coronary heart disease. *Indian Heart J.*, 2016 Jul-Aug, *68*(4), 498-506. doi: 10.1016/j.ihj.2015.10.384.

[3] Gopalakrishnan, S., Mathew, P. & Vaidyanathan, K. (2017). Attitude of Bachelor of Dental Surgery students and interns toward teaching-learning process in Government Dental College, Kottayam, Kerala, India. Indian J Dent Res. 28(3):256-260. doi: 10.4103/ijdr.IJDR_ 121_16.

[4] Vaidyanathan, K. & Gopalakrishnan, S. (2017). Nanomedicine in the diagnosis and treatment of atherosclerosis – A systematic review.

Cardiovasc Hematol Disord Drug Targets., *17*(2), 119-131. doi: 10.2174/1871529X17666170918142653. PMID: 28925905.

[5] Vaidyanathan, K. & Gopalakrishnan, S. (2018). Novel biomarkers for inborn errors of metabolism in the metabolomics era. *Indian Journal of Biochemistry & Biophysics*, NISCAIR-CSIR, 2018 (Accepted for publication).

[6] Varghese, R., Dalvi, Y. B., Nair, C. K. K. & Vaidyanathan, K. (2018). Toxicological Evaluation and Oral Glucose Tolerance Test Of Ganoderma Applanatum (Pers.) Pat. From Kerala. Research *Journal of Life Sciences, Bioinformatics, Pharmaceutical and Chemical Sciences, RJLBPCS*, 2018 (Accepted for publication).

In: Horizons in Cancer Research. Volume 73 ISBN: 978-1-53616-273-8
Editor: Hiroto S. Watanabe

Chapter 3

RAD51 Is Involved in Cisplatin Resistance in Ovarian Cancer

Guanhua Qian and Tinghe Yu*
Key Medical Laboratory of Obstetrics and Gynecology, The Second Affiliated Hospital, Chongqing Medical University, Chongqing, China

Abstract

Cancer commonly has a high level of DNA replication, damage and repair. RAD51 plays an important role in homologous recombination, a pathway of DNA repair. Recent data have manifested that RAD51 is involved in platinum resistance in ovarian cancer. Platinum agents induce DNA breaks; therefore, DNA repair may lead to cell survival, and eventually results in treatment failure. Here underlying mechanisms are discussed in brief. Further, RAD51 is a potential target to manage chemoresistant cancers. Certain drugs and strategies can sensitize chemotherapy via impacting on RAD51, which can be developed as chemotherapy modulators.

Keywords: RAD51, DNA repair, chemoresistance, cisplatin

---

* Corresponding Author's Email: yutinghe@hotmail.com.

1. Introduction

RAD51, as a DNA repair gene, plays an important role in maintenance of the gene stability via involving in homologous recombination (HR). The abnormal expression of RAD51 is closely related to the occurrence, development and treatment tolerance of certain cancers.

Ovarian cancer has the highest mortality among gynecological malignances [1]. The occurrence of ovarian cancer is a complex multi-gene and -stage process, during which the malfunction of DNA repair leads to chromosome aberration and gene mutations contributing to the occurrence and progression of cancer. Cytoreductive surgery followed by chemotherapy has been the standard regimen. Platinum-based chemotherapy is the first-line regimen. However, drug resistance will gradually emerge during treatments, and ultimately leads to treatment failure [2]. Therefore, overcoming resistance can improve the clinical outcome [3].

HR, as a DNA repair mechanism, has a high validity and accuracy, and plays an important role in maintenance of the genome stability and physiological functions [4, 5]. RAD51 is a key protein of HR. Platinum agents deactivate cancer cells mainly via inducing DNA damages, and those unrepairable cells usually undergo apoptosis and/or necrosis. Therefore, RAD51 plays a critical role in platinum resistance. Recently, RAD51 is considered a target for overcoming drug resistance. Here the role of RAD51 in platinum resistance in ovarian cancer is briefly discussed.

2. Structure and Function of RAD51

2.1. Structure of RAD51

The length of human RAD51 gene is 30 kb with 9 exons and 8 introns, encoding a protein consisting of 339 amino acids. It locates at 15q15.1 [6]. XRCC2, XRCC3, RAD51B (RAD51L1), RAD51C (RAD51L2) and RAD51D (RAD51L3) are homologues of RAD51, and participate in HR with RAD51 [7].

2.2. Biological Function of RAD51

DNA double-strand break (DSB) can be directly induced by ionizing radiation, alkylating agents, topoisomerase II inhibitors and hypoxia, or is a result of exacerbation of single-strand break (SSB). DSB can lead to permanent arrest of cell cycle, thereby endangering the cell survival. HR and non-homologous end joining (NHEJ) are the two mechanisms to repair DSB, and HR is the main pathway in eukaryotes [8-10]. Most importantly, HR can realize error-free repair [11].

RAD51 promotes the chain exchange and homologous pairing, and participates in DNA damage reactions. Repairing spontaneous DNA damages depends on appropriate expression of RAD51. Knocking-out of RAD51 results in death of mouse embryo [12]. A high expression level of RAD51 can contribute to the tumor progression, and drug/radiation resistance by causing genomic instability [13]. The overexpression of RAD51 is detected in certain human tumors such as cancers of breast, lung and ovary, suggesting that high expression of RAD51 can be a biomarker to predict the response to chemotherapy or radiotherapy.

3. Mechanisms of Resistance to Cisplatin

Mechanisms of cisplatin (DDP) resistance include the decrease of intracellular drug accumulation, drug inactivation, improvement of DNA repair, and apoptotic malfunction.

3.1. Drug Accumulation and Inactivation

Drug influx and efflux determine the intracellular drug level. The influx of DDP is mediated by passive diffusion and the copper transporter (CTR1). The weight of each pathway depends on cell type. Passive diffusion is mainly determined by membrane fluidity [14]. Rigid cell membranes with a high level of sphingomyelin and cholesterol lower the DDP uptake in resistant cells [15, 16]. Certain drugs such as dinitrophenol, in combination with NaF or iodoacetate, can decrease DDP accumulation via modulating the property of cell membrane. Moreover, DDP itself can affect certain membrane properties, resulting in acquired resistance [17, 18]. CTR1 mediates the active uptake of DDP. Knockdown of CTR1 in fibroblasts in mouse embryo decreases DDP accumulation [19, 20]. Therefore, CTR1 is a determinant of DDP sensitivity in certain cells [21, 22]. The decrease of DDP uptake can also be attributed to other factors, including folates, epidermal growth factor (EGF), iron, glucose, etc. [23].

The copper-transporting P-type ATPase ATP7A and ATP7B are implicated in platinum efflux and resistance [24-30]. The expression level of ATP7A and ATP7B is up-regulated in certain DDP-resistant cells [31, 32], and over-expression of ATP7A promotes the drug efflux resulting in resistance [30]. Clinical data have manifested that the expression level of ATP7B can predict the DDP sensitivity in ovarian cancer cells [33]. The metallochaperone protein Atox1 is associated with DDP resistance. Atox1 regulates DDP uptake by modulating the function of CTR1. Loss of Atox1 decreases the uptake and intracellular accumulation of DDP [34].

Chemoresistance can occur when the cellular processes of DDP are impeded. Glutathione (GSH) can bind with DDP and decrease its activity, which can lead to DDP resistance. DDP-GSH complexes are formed under the catalysis of glutathione-S-transferase (GST) [35, 36]. This mechanism has been clinically noted [37]. Gamma-glutamyltransferase (GGT) can catalyze the synthesis of GSH, and over-expression of GGT is involved in DDP resistance [38]. Metallothioneins play a part in DDP resistance through drug binding [39]. The expression level of metallothionein is positively correlated with the DDP response in ovarian cancer [40].

3.2. DNA Repair Systems

DDP-induced DNA damages can be repaired via nucleotide excision repair (NER), mismatch repair (MMR) or HR. The process of NER consists of identification of DNA damage, excision of DNA damages and DNA synthesis at the excised site. ERCC1, as an endonuclease related to NER, is a determinant of therapeutic efficacy to platinum-based regimen in ovarian cancer [41]. ERCC1 also participates in repair of interstrand-crosslink repair (ICR) attributable to DDP [42-44]. Noticeably, overexpression of ERCC1 does not necessarily lead to DDP resistance. Transfection of ERCC1 improves the DDP sensitivity in hamster ovarian cells [45]. This may relate to the imbalance among DNA repair pathways.

MMR may lead to apoptosis, and is related to platinum sensitivity [46]. A decrease of MMR proteins MLH1, MSH2 or MSH6, increases DDP resistance [47-49]. Deficiency of MMR is accompanied with a decrease in microsatellite instability and apoptosis [48, 50], leading to DDP resistance.

BRCA1, BRCA2 and RAD51 are three critical components in HR. Ovarian cancer with BRCA1/2 deficiency is more sensitive to platinum in compassion with cancer without deficiency [51, 52]. In sensitive tumors with BRCA2 defections, tumors gradually become resistant to DDP [53, 54] after BRCA2 mutations, which is related to the recovery of HR. RAD51 catalyzes the exchange of homologous DNA strands. RAD51 is with a high expression level in certain tumors, increasing DNA repair capacity to lead to tolerance to radiotherapy and chemotherapy.

3.3. Apoptosis Pathway

DDP induces apoptosis through the Fas/Fas ligand and/or mitochondrial pathways [55]. P53 is a key protein in apoptosis, and is essential for DDP-induced apoptosis [56-58]. It is reported that cancers with wild-type p53 expression are more likely to achieve better therapeutic outcome compared with cancers with p53 mutations [59, 60].

The signaling transport of DDP-apoptosis is not well known. The DDP sensitivity in ovarian cancer cells depends on the persistent activation of SAPK/JNK and p38 kinases, as well as the successive activation of AP-1 and FasL [61]. In DDP-resistant cells, SAPK/JNK signaling pathway is only temporarily activated and FasL apoptosis signal is lack [62].

4. RAD51 in Cancer Chemoresistance

DNA repair occurs frequently during cancer progression, which leads to accumulation of genetic defects, thereby facilitating rapid evolution of the tumor cell population and promoting intrinsic resistance to DNA-damaging agents [63].

Overexpression of RAD51 increases the HR capacity and gene instability [64]. RAD51 gene loses heterozygosity and is with a high expression level in many cancer types, such as breast, pancreas, ovary and colorectum [13]. RAD51 is up-regulated in lung cancer in comparison with normal tissues, and a high expression level is associated with poor survival [65].

DDP can cause DSB and inhibit DNA synthesis, eventually leading to cell death [66]. An improvement of DNA repair capacity frequently results in chemotherapy resistance. HR is the main mode of DSB repair [67].

DDP resistance attributable to RAD51 is related to BRCA1 and BRCA2. RAD51 can arrest cell cycle through BRCA1, and then repair DNA with the assistance of BRCA2. BRCA2 regulates the function of RAD51 via binding with RAD51. The signals of DNA damages activate certain kinases (e.g., ATM, ATR), thereby catalyzing the BRCA2/RAD51 complex phosphorylation to generate the active form. BRCA2/RAD51 complex transports to the DSB site and participates in recombination of dsDNA [68, 69]. Further, DDP can induce the expression of RAD51 to enhance DNA repair. Silencing BRCA2 can suppress the expression of BRCA2 and RAD51, decrease DNA repair and enhance the action of DDP. The expression level of RAD51, BRCA1 and BRCA 2 is correlated with the therapeutic response to DDP-based regimen in ovarian cancer. Patients with a low expression level of BRCA1/BRCA2 in cancer tissues have longer survival time [70].

5. Strategies to Target RAD51

The role of RAD51 in HR demonstrates a therapeutic target. Those strategies utilize nucleotide or chemical components (e.g., siRNA and small molecules) that can inhibit the expression or function of RAD5, thereby sensitizing antitumor drugs to improve the therapeutic outcome.

5.1. RNA Interference (RNAi)

5.1.1. Direct Regulation

RNAi can specifically inhibit gene expression by impairing the transcription or translation, using small interference RNA (siRNA) or microRNA (miRNA). RAD51 knockdown by siRNA can increase the cells' sensitivity to anticancer drugs [71]. The sensitization is not observed in normal human fibroblasts. These data indicate that the effect of suppressing RAD51 on DDP sensitivity varies between cancer and cell types. In vivo trials have manifested that inhibiting RAD51 with siRNA can increase the drug sensitivity and suppress tumor growth [72]. Chemotherapy sensitization attributable to down-knocking RAD51 is even detected in cancer stem cells [73].

miRNA is a class of small non-coding RNAs that regulates gene function. A low expression level of RAD51 regulation miRNA (miR-506) corresponds with drug resistance and tumor relapse in ovarian cancer, indicating that miR-506 can be a prognosis marker and a therapeutic target [74]. Injecting miR-506 can increase the sensitivity to DDP in mice bearing ovarian tumors. miR-506 impairs the RAD51 gene expression by directly binding to RAD51 dsDNA. Additionally, miR-34s family (miR-34a, miR-34b, miR-34c, and miR-34-5p) can bind with the RAD51 mRNA 3'-UTR to suppress the expression of RAD51 [75]. Data have demonstrated that miRNAs can directly inhibit the expression of RAD51: miR-96 targets the coding region of RAD51 [76]; and miR-155, miR-103 and miR-107 target the 3'-UTR of RAD51 [77, 78]. These miRNAs may be employed to reverse chemoresistance.

Short hairpin RNA (shRNA) is similar with siRNA but contains a hairpin structure that connects the sense and anti-sense strands. shRNA can be transmitted into cells using the virus vector. shRNA can generate sustained siRNA expression, thus realizing prolonged gene silence [79]. Suppression of RAD51 with shRNA leads to G2 arrest, thereby inhibiting cell proliferation increasing the sensitivity to DDP [80, 81].

5.1.2. Indirect Interference

Certain strategies utilize siRNA or miRNA that does not directly inhibit the expression of RAD51. These molecules inhibit the expression of related genes, and subsequently impair the expression of RAD51 or affect its biological function. miR-99 family can target SNF2H, a SWI/SNF chromatin remodeling factor, resulting in a deficiency of RAD51 recruitment to the DNA damage site [82]. Nucleolin is involved in regulation of resistance to replication stress due to antitumor drugs. Down-regulating the expression of nucleolin with siRNA reduces the formation of RAD51 foci, thereby suppressing HR [83]. Certain proteins can affect the accumulation of RAD51 to the DNA break site.

Cyclin D1 is also responsible for the formation of RAD51 foci [84]. Using siRNA to inhibit the expression of Cyclin D1 can decrease the RAD51 foci. Further, down-regulation of Cyclin D1 can induce G0/G1 arrest, and therefore HR cannot be initiated. Consequently, the drug sensitivity is increased and a better therapeutic outcome is realized.

The inhibition of KIF4A by siRNA enhances the action of DDP. KIF4A is required for RAD51 recruitment. The KIF4A depletion can inhibit RAD51 recruitment induced by radiation, thereby impairing HR [85].

5.2. Small Molecule Inhibitors

The formation of RAD51 foci that binds to single-stranded DNA (ssDNA) is required for initiating HR. Certain small molecules that can inhibit the binding of RAD51 to ssDNA have been identified in recent years. Takako et al. screened 185 chemical compounds, and found that 4,4'-

diisothiocyanostilbene-2,2'-disulfonic acid (DIDS) can inhibit the RAD51-mediated strand exchange [86]. DIDS competes with RAD51 to bind DNA, thereby impairing HR. DIDS alone or combined with other chemicals to interfere with RAD51 can increase the drug sensitivity [87-89].

Metatungstate is another RAD51 inhibitor. Metatungstate can disturb the function of MvRadA, a homologue of RAD51. Metatungstate can inhibite the ssDNA binding, strand exchange and ATPase activity, and can lock RAD protein to the inactive form [90]. Fluorescence resonance energy transfer (FRET) is recently employed to assay the interaction between a molecule and the target site, thereby screening active molecules. Huang et al. developed a FRET-based assay and screened about 200000 small molecules from the NIH Small Molecule Repository [91]. 17 chemicals were identified, and the compound B02 exhibited the activity of RAD51 inhibition by impeding DNA strand exchange. B02 directly binds to RAD51 to inhibit its binding to ssDNA [92]. In vivo data have demonstrated a reduction of tumor growth due to DDP, after inhibiting RAD51 with B02 [93].

RI-1 can specifically inhibit RAD51 by interrupting the formation of RAD51-ssDNA [94]. The chloromaleimide group of RI-1 can function as a Michael acceptor, and inhibit RAD51 by binding to the Cys319 residue. RI-1 can prevent oligomerization of RAD51 into filaments on DNA.

2-(benzylsulfonyl)-1-(1H-indol-3-yl)-1,2-dihydroisoquinoline (IRB2) can inhibit the function of RAD51 [95], which disrupts the RAD51 multimerization and accelerates proteasome-mediated RAD51 degradation by mimicking BRC. IRB2 directly binds to RAD51 and prevents the foci formation, displaying a broad-spectrum anti-proliferation capability. Chicago Sky Blue can prevent the binding of RAD51 to ssDNA, and therefore inhibits the subsequent strand exchange [96].

The interruption of RAD51 binding to ssDNA impairs HR. RAD51 is also a key protein in maintenance of replication forks in normal cells. Therefore, interrupting RAD51 binding may affect highly proliferative normal cells such as bone marrow cells, resulting in undesired toxicity [97]. The D-loop formation in HR may be an alternative target. When binding with ssDNA, RAD51 promotes the identification of homologous sequence in dsDNA, and creates a joint structure that consists of a heteroduplex and a displaced strand of ssDNA (D-loop); the DNA synthesis is initiated using the formed homologous strand as the template [98]. The second class of inhibitors can specifically prevent the RAD51-mediated D-loop formation, whilst preserving its binding capability with ssDNA. Halenaquinone, which is the oncogenic protein tyrosine kinase encoded by the Aous sarcoma virus, can inhibit pp60v-src [99]. Takaku et al. identified halenaquinone as a RAD51 inhibitor [100]. Halenaquinone can inhibit the secondary RAD51-dsDNA binding and the D-loop formation, but not affect the RAD51-ssDNA binding. Halenaquinone can decrease the retention time of RAD51 at the DSB site.

Lv et al. performed a two-part high-throughput (HT) screen of the ASDI diversity library and LOPAC1280 compound library, and identified a compound that can specifically inhibit D-loop while having minimal effect on RAD51-ssDNA. The oxidized form of this compound (i.e., RI(dl)-1) can inhibit the D-loop formation [101]. The IC_{50} of RI(dl)-1 is 13.0 μM. Modifying the structure of RI(dl)-1 leads to the discovery RI(dl)-2. RI(dl)-2 has an enhanced anti-D-loop formation capability (with IC_{50} of 11.1 μM) without effects on RAD51-ssDNA binding. RI(dl)-2 may be the first compound that can specifically inhibit the D-loop formation.

Many factors regulate the expression and/or the biological function of RAD51. The tyrosine kinases BRC-ABL and c-ABL up-regulate the expression of RAD51, improving HR to result in drug-resistance. Therefore, tyrosine kinases can be the targets for RAD51. Anti-leukemia agent imatinib is an inhibitor of c-ABL. Delayed tumor growth due to imatinib is related to a decrease of RAD51 expression after inhibiting c-ABL, and imatinib can also increase the chemosensitivity [102]. Amuvatinib, icotinib and gefitinib can modulate RAD51 expression, thereby increasing chemosensitivity via decreasing HR [103-105]

Another widely used indirect target is the histone deacetylase. Histone deacetylase removes the acetyl groups from N-acetyl lysine amino acid on histone, and is involved in the post-translational modification of histone and non-histone acetylation, thus influencing gene expression [106]. Delivery of the histone deacetylase inhibitor MS-275 into tumor xenografts affects several proteins, including down-regulation of RAD51 [107]. Panobinostat inhibits the activity of histone deacetylase, thereby subsequently suppressing expression of BRCA1, CHK1 and RAD51 [108]. Data in a xenograft model have demonstrated that panobinostat enhances the chemosensitivity. Chemosensitization is also observed in other histone deacetylase inhibitors such as vorinostat, PCI-24781 and suberoylanilidehydroxamic acid (SAHA) [109-111].

Our data have manifested that thioridazine, as an antischizophrenic drug, can inhibit human cancer cells of uterine cervix, lung and ovary [112-114]. Thioridazine induced cell death, and the combination of thioridazine and DDP led to the highest percentage of dead cells in A549, A549/DDP, SKOV3 and SKOV3/DDP cells, where A549/DDP and SKOV3/DDP were chemoresistant sublines. Thioridazine and the combined modality led to cell apoptosis via inducing G0/G1 arrest, resulting in mitochondria dependent apoptosis. These data indicated that thioridazine can sensitize DDP. Cytotoxicity of DDP is mostly mediated by DNA damages [115]. Most present chemotherapy modulators sensitize DDP via inhibiting DNA repair [116]. Thioridazine with a high concentration can cause DNA damages and has anti-proliferative activity [113, 114, 117, 118]. Therefore, Thio may impact on RAD51 to impair DNA repair.

5.3. Nanotechnology in the Delivery of RAD51 Inhibitors

Nanotechnology has been emerged as a new therapeutic strategy. Incorporating drugs or RNAs into nano vesicles can enhance the tumor targeting. Tatyana et al. incorporated RAD51 siRNA into exosomes which were delivered into cancer cells [119]. This modality enhanced the cellular uptake and gene-silencing capability. The findings demonstrated the role of exosome in augmentation of the gene-silencing capability. Yu et al. constructed Ag/C225 nanoparticles which consisted of silver nanoparticles and the anti-growth factor receptor antibody C225. Nanoparticles inhibited the expression of DNA repair genes including RAD51 [120]. Meena et al. prepared PLGA nanoparticles loaded curcumin. Data showed that these nanoparticles increased the cellular uptake, and that the expression of DNA repair genes were suppressed such as BRCA1, BRCA2 and RAD51 [121]. Iron-oxide nanoparticles (MN-OA) can target HSP90 and down-regulate the expression of RAD51 [122].

Conclusion

RAD51 plays a crucial role in the occurrence, progression and therapeutic tolerance of ovarian cancer. RAD51 can be a target for cancer treatments. Certain strategies have been in progress, and may be utilized to modulate DDP-based chemotherapy and to overcome chemotherapy resistance.

References

[1] Jemal A, Bray F, Center MM, et al. Global cancer statistics. *CA Cancer J Clin* 2011, 61: 69-90.

[2] Shih KK, Chi DS. Maximal cytoreductive effort in epithelial ovarian cancer surgery. *J Gynecol Oncol* 2010, 21: 75-80.

[3] Koberle B, Tomicic MT, Usanova S, et al. Cisplatin resistance: preclinical findings and clinical implications. *Biochim Biophys Acta* 2010, 1806:172-182.

[4] Kakarougkas A, Jeggo PA. DNA DSB repair pathway choice: an orchestrated handover mechanism. *Br J Radiol* 2014, 87: 20130685.

[5] Srivastava M, Raghavan SC. DNA double-strand break repair inhibitors as cancer therapeutics. *Chem Biol* 2015, 22: 17-29.

[6] Shinohara A, Ogawa H, Matsuda Y, et al. Cloning of human, mouse and fission yeast recombination genes homologous to RAD51 and recA. *Nat Genet* 1993, 4: 239-243.

[7] Taylor M, Spirek M, Chaurasiya KR, et al. Rad51 paralogs remodel pre-synaptic Rad51 filaments to stimulate homologous recombination. *Cell* 2015, 162: 271-286.

[8] Gonzalez F, Georgieva D, Vanoli F, et al. Homologous recombination DNA repair genes play a critical role in reprogramming to a pluripotent state. *Cell Rep* 2013, 3: 651-660.

[9] Felgentreff K, Du L, Weinacht KG, et al. Differential role of nonhomologous end joining factors in the generation, DNA damage response, and myeloid differentiation of human induced pluripotent stem cells. *Proc Natl Acad Sci USA* 2014, 111: 8889-8894.

[10] Ciccia A, Elledge SJ. The DNA damage response: making it safe to play with knives. *Mol Cell* 2010, 40: 179-204.

[11] Miyagawa K. Clinical relevance of the homologous recombination machinery in cancer therapy. *Cancer Sci* 2008, 99: 187-194.

[12] Richardson C, Stark JM, Ommundsen M, et al. M. Rad51 overexpression promotes alternative double-strand break repair pathways and genome instability. *Oncogene* 2004, 23: 546-553.

[13] Klein HL. The consequences of Rad51 overexpression for normal and tumor cells. *DNA Repair* 2008, 7: 686-693.

[14] Mann SC, Andrews PA, Howell SB. Comparison of lipid content, surface membrane fluidity, and temperature dependence of cis-diamminedichloroplatinum(II) accumulation in sensitive and resistant human ovarian carcinoma cells. *Anticancer Res* 1988, 8: 1211-1215.

[15] Popovic P, Goel R, Evans WK, et al. Pressure-tuning infrared spectra of cisplatin sensitive and resistant human ovarian cancer cells exposed to cisplatin. *Proc Am Assoc Cancer Res* 1993, 34: 404.

[16] Popovic P, Kates M, Grewaal D, et al. Membrane fluidity and lipids in cisplatin resistant cells with low cisplatin uptake. *Proc Am Assoc Cancer Res* 1994, 35: 440.

[17] Sdjppmjmmnzmhg R. Effect of cations on cisplatin uptake and efficacy in lung cancer cell lines. *Proc Am Asso Cancer Res* 1995, 36: 399.

[18] Andrews PA, Velury S, Mann SC, et al. cis-Diamminedichloroplatinum(II) accumulation in sensitive and resistant human ovarian carcinoma cells. *Cancer Res* 1988, 48: 68-73.

[19] Ishida S, Lee J, Thiele DJ, et al. Uptake of the anticancer drug cisplatin mediated by the copper transporter Ctr1 in yeast and mammals. *Proc Natl Acad Sci USA* 2002, 99: 14298-14302.

[20] Holzer AK, Manorek MG, Howell SB. Contribution of the major copper influx transporter CTR1 to the cellular accumulation of cisplatin, carboplatin, and oxaliplatin. *Mol Pharmacol* 2006, 70: 1390-1394.

[21] Song IS, Savaraj N, Siddik ZH, et al. Role of human copper transporter Ctr1 in the transport of platinum-based antitumor agents in cisplatin-sensitive and cisplatin-resistant cells. *Mol Cancer Ther* 2004, 3: 1543-1549.

[22] Min Y, Mao C, Chen S, et al. Combating the drug resistance of cisplatin using a platinum prodrug based delivery system. *Angew Chem Int Ed Engl* 2012, 51: 6742-6747.

[23] Shen DW, Su A, Liang XJ, et al. Reduced expression of small GTPases and hypermethylation of the folate binding protein gene in cisplatin-resistant cells. *Br J Cancer* 2004, 91: 270-276.

[24] Safaei R, Katano K, Samimi G, et al. Cross-resistance to cisplatin in cells with acquired resistance to copper. *Cancer Chemother Pharmacol* 2004, 53: 239-246.

[25] Nakayama K, Miyazaki K, Kanzaki A, et al. Expression and cisplatin sensitivity of copper-transporting P-type adenosine triphosphatase (ATP7B) in human solid carcinoma cell lines. *Oncol Rep* 2001, 8: 1285-1287.

[26] Katano K, Safaei R, Samimi G, et al. The copper export pump ATP7B modulates the cellular pharmacology of carboplatin in ovarian carcinoma cells. *Mol Pharmacol* 2003, 64: 466-473.

[27] Higashimoto M, Kanzaki A, Shimakawa T, et al. Expression of copper-transporting P-type adenosine triphosphatase in human esophageal carcinoma. *Int J Mol Med* 2003, 11: 337-341.

[28] Miyashita H, Nitta Y, Mori S, et al. Expression of copper-transporting P-type adenosine triphosphatase (ATP7B) as a chemoresistance marker in human oral squamous cell carcinoma treated with cisplatin. *Oral Oncol* 2003, 39: 157-162.

[29] Safaei R, Larson BJ, Cheng TC, et al. Abnormal lysosomal trafficking and enhanced exosomal export of cisplatin in drug-resistant human ovarian carcinoma cells. *Mol Cancer Ther* 2005, 4: 1595-1604.

[30] Samimi G, Safaei R, Katano K, et al. Increased expression of the copper efflux transporter ATP7A mediates resistance to cisplatin, carboplatin, and oxaliplatin in ovarian cancer cells. *Clin Cancer Res* 2004, 10: 4661-4669.

[31] Safaei R, Holzer AK, Katano K, et al. The role of copper transporters in the development of resistance to Pt drugs. *J Inorg Biochem* 2004, 98: 1607-1613.

[32] Dmitriev OY. Mechanism of tumor resistance to cisplatin mediated by the copper transporter ATP7B. *Biochem Cell Biol* 2011, 89: 138-147.

[33] Nakayama K, Kanzaki A, Ogawa K, et al. Copper-transporting P-type adenosine triphosphatase (ATP7B) as a cisplatin based chemoresistance marker in ovarian carcinoma: comparative analysis with expression of MDR1, MRP1, MRP2, LRP and BCRP. *Int J Cancer* 2002, 101: 488-495.

[34] Safaei R, Maktabi MH, Blair BG, et al. Effects of the loss of Atox1 on the cellular pharmacology of cisplatin. *J Inorg Biochem* 2009, 103: 333-341.

[35] Goto S, Iida T, Cho S, et al. Overexpression of glutathione S-transferase pi enhances the adduct formation of cisplatin with glutathione in human cancer cells. *Free Radic Res* 1999, 31: 549-558.

[36] Shoeib T, Sharp B. Monomeric cisplatin complexes with glutathione: coordination modes and binding affinities. *Inorg Chim Acta* 2013, 405: 258–264.

[37] Sakamoto M, Kondo A, Kawasaki K, et al. Analysis of gene expression profiles associated with cisplatin resistance in human ovarian cancer cell lines and tissues using cDNA microarray. *Human Cell* 2001, 14: 305-315.

[38] Daubeuf S, Leroy P, Paolicchi A, et al. Enhanced resistance of HeLa cells to cisplatin by overexpression of gamma-glutamyltransferase. *Biochem Pharmacol* 2002, 64: 207-216.

[39] Zhang GX, Hu W, Wang FY. A comparative study on interactions of cisplatin and ruthenium arene anticancer complexes with metallothionein using MALDI-TOF-MS. *Int J Mass Spectrom* 2011, 307: 79-84.

[40] Surowiak P, Materna V, Maciejczyk A, et al. Nuclear metallothionein expression correlates with cisplatin resistance of ovarian cancer cells and poor clinical outcome. *Virchows Archiv* 2007, 450: 279-285.

[41] Dabholkar M, Bostick-Bruton F, Weber C, et al. ERCC1 and ERCC2 expression in malignant tissues from ovarian cancer patients. *J Natl Cancer Inst* 1992, 84: 1512-1517.

[42] Niedernhofer LJ, Odijk H, Budzowska M, et al. The structure-specific endonuclease Ercc1-Xpf is required to resolve DNA interstrand cross-link-induced double-strand breaks. *Mol Cell Biol* 2004, 24: 5776-5787.

[43] Usanova S, Piee-Staffa A, Sied U, et al. Cisplatin sensitivity of testis tumour cells is due to deficiency in interstrand-crosslink repair and low ERCC1-XPF expression. *Mol Cancer* 2010, 9: 248.

[44] Zhen W, Link CJ, O'Connor PM, et al. Increased gene-specific repair of cisplatin interstrand cross-links in cisplatin-resistant human ovarian cancer cell lines. *Mol Cell Biol* 1992, 12: 3689-3698.

[45] Bramson J, Panasci LC. Effect of ERCC1 overexpression on sensitivity of chinese-hamster ovary cells to DNA-damaging agents. *Cancer Res* 1993, 53: 3237-3240.

[46] Berry SE, Kinsella TJ. Targeting DNA mismatch repair for radiosensitization. *Semin Radiat Oncol* 2001, 11: 300-315.

[47] Lage H, Christmann M, Kern MA, et al. Expression of DNA repair proteins hMSH2, hMSH6, hMLH1, O6-methylguanine-DNA methyltransferase and N-methylpurine-DNA glycosylase in melanoma cells with acquired drug resistance. *Int J Cancer* 1999, 80: 744-750.

[48] Anthoney DA, Mcllwrath AJ, Gallagher WM, et al. Microsatellite instability, apoptosis, and loss of p53 function in drug-resistant tumor cells. *Cancer Res* 1996, 56: 1374-1381.

[49] Vaisman A, Varchenko M, Umar A, et al. The role of hMLH1, hMSH3, and hMSH6 defects in cisplatin and oxaliplatin resistance: correlation with replicative bypass of platinum-DNA adducts. *Cancer Res* 1998, 58: 3579-3585.

[50] Mayer F, Gillis AJ, Dinjens W, et al. Microsatellite instability of germ cell tumors is associated with resistance to systemic treatment. *Cancer Res* 2002, 62: 2758-2760.

[51] Chetrit A, Hirsh-Yechezkel G, Ben-David Y, et al. Effect of BRCA1/2 mutations on long-term survival of patients with invasive ovarian cancer: the national Israeli study of ovarian cancer. *J Clin Oncol* 2008, 26: 20-25.

[52] Gourley C, Michie CO, Roxburgh P, et al. Increased incidence of visceral metastases in scottish patients with BRCA1/2-defective ovarian cancer: an extension of the ovarian BRCAness phenotype. *J Clin Oncol* 2010, 28: 2505-2511.

[53] Edwards SL, Brough R, Lord CJ, et al. Resistance to therapy caused by intragenic deletion in BRCA2. *Nature* 2008, 451: 1111-1115.

[54] Sakai W, Swisher EM, Karlan BY, et al. Secondary mutations as a mechanism of cisplatin resistance in BRCA2-mutated cancers. *Nature* 2008, 451: 1116-1120.

[55] Gonzalez VM, Fuertes MA, Alonso C, et al. Is cisplatin-induced cell death always produced by apoptosis? *Mol Pharmacol* 2001, 59: 657-663.

[56] Branch P, Masson M, Aquilina G, et al. Spontaneous development of drug resistance: mismatch repair and p53 defects in resistance to cisplatin in human tumor cells. *Oncogene* 2000, 19: 3138-3145.

[57] Hengstler JG, Pilch H, Schmidt M, et al. Metallothionein expression in ovarian cancer in relation to histopathological parameters and molecular markers of prognosis. *Int J Cancer* 2001, 95: 121-127.

[58] Kim CW, Lu JN, Go SI, et al. p53 restoration can overcome cisplatin resistance through inhibition of Akt as well as induction of Bax. *Int J Oncol* 2013, 43: 1495-1502.
[59] Gadducci A, Cosio S, Muraca S, et al. Molecular mechanisms of apoptosis and chemosensitivity to platinum and paclitaxel in ovarian cancer: biological data and clinical implications. *Eur J Gynaecol Oncol* 2002, 23: 390-396.
[60] Feldman DR, Bosl GJ, Sheinfeld J, et al. Medical treatment of advanced testicular cancer. *JAMA* 2008, 299: 672-684.
[61] Mansouri A, Ridgway LD, Korapati AL, et al. Sustained activation of JNK/p38 MAPK pathways in response to cisplatin leads to Fas ligand induction and cell death in ovarian carcinoma cells. *J Biol Chem* 2003, 278: 19245-19256.
[62] Brozovic A, Fritz G, Christmann M, et al. Long-term activation of SAPK/JNK, p38 kinase and fas-L expression by cisplatin is attenuated in human carcinoma cells that acquired drug resistance. *Int J Cancer* 2004, 112: 974-985.
[63] Harris JL, Rabellino A, Khanna KK. RAD51 paralogs promote genomic integrity and chemoresistance in cancer by facilitating homologous recombination. *Ann Transl Med* 2018, 6: S122.
[64] Richardson C, Stark JM, Ommundsen M, et al. Rad51 overexpression promotes alternative double-strand break repair pathways and genome instability. *Oncogene* 2004, 23: 546-553.
[65] Hu J, Zhang Z, Zhao L, et al. High expression of RAD51 promotes DNA damage repair and survival in KRAS-mutant lung cancer cells. *BMB Rep* 2019, 52: 151-156.
[66] Yan D, An G, Kuo MT. C-Jun N-terminal kinase signalling pathway in response to cisplatin. *J Cell Mol Med* 2016, 20: 2013-2019.
[67] Gavande NS, VanderVere-Carozza PS, Hinshaw HD, et al. DNA repair targeted therapy: the past or future of cancer treatment? *Pharmacol Ther* 2016, 160: 65-83.
[68] Cousineau I, Belmaaza A. EMSY overexpression disrupts the BRCA2/RAD51 pathway in the DNA-damage response: implications

for chromosomal instability/recombination syndromes as checkpoint diseases. *Mol Genet Genomics* 2011, 285: 325-340.

[69] Nogueira A, Catarino R, Coelho A, et al. Influence of DNA repair RAD51 gene variants in overall survival of non-small cell lung cancer patients treated with first line chemotherapy. *Cancer Chemother Pharmacol* 2010, 66: 501-506.

[70] Wan B, Dai L, Wang L, et al. Knockdown of BRCA2 enhances cisplatin and cisplatin-induced autophagy in ovarian cancer cells. *Endocr Relat Cancer* 2018, 25: 69-82.

[71] Ito M, Yamamoto S, Nimura K, et al. Rad51 siRNA delivered by HVJ envelope vector enhances the anti-cancer effect of cisplatin. *J Gene Med* 2005, 7: 1044-1052.

[72] Kiyohara E, Tamai K, Katayama I, et al. The combination of chemotherapy with HVJ-E containing Rad51 siRNA elicited diverse anti-tumor effects and synergistically suppressed melanoma. *Gene Ther* 2012, 19: 734-741.

[73] Ruiz G, Valencia-Gonzalez HA, Leon-Galicia I, et al. Inhibition of RAD51 by siRNA and resveratrol sensitizes cancer stem cells derived from HeLa cell cultures to apoptosis. *Stem Cells Int* 2018, 2018: 2493869.

[74] Liu G, Yang D, Rupaimoole R, et al. Augmentation of response to chemotherapy by microRNA-506 through regulation of RAD51 in serous ovarian cancers. *J Natl Cancer Inst* 2015, 107: djv108 .

[75] Chen S, Liu R, Wang Q, et al. MiR-34s negatively regulate homologous recombination through targeting RAD51. *Arch Biochem Biophys* 2019, 666: 73-82.

[76] Wang Y, Huang JW, Calses P, et al. MiR-96 downregulates REV1 and RAD51 to promote cellular sensitivity to cisplatin and PARP inhibition. *Cancer Res* 2012, 72: 4037-4046.

[77] Gasparini P, Lovat F, Fassan M, et al. Protective role of miR-155 in breast cancer through RAD51 targeting impairs homologous recombination after irradiation. *Proc Natl Acad Sci USA* 2014, 111: 4536-4541.

[78] Huang JW, Wang Y, Dhillon KK, et al. Systematic screen identifies miRNAs that target RAD51 and RAD51D to enhance chemosensitivity. *Mol Cancer Res* 2013, 11: 1564-1573.

[79] Rossi JJ. Expression strategies for short hairpin RNA interference triggers. *Hum Gene Ther* 2008, 19: 313-317.

[80] Quiros S, Roos WP, Kaina B. Rad51 and BRCA2--New molecular targets for sensitizing glioma cells to alkylating anticancer drugs. *PloS One* 2011, 6: e27183.

[81] Du LQ, Wang Y, Wang H, et al. Knockdown of Rad51 expression induces radiation- and chemo-sensitivity in osteosarcoma cells. *Med Oncol* 2011, 28: 1481-1487.

[82] Mueller AC, Sun D, Dutta A. The miR-99 family regulates the DNA damage response through its target SNF2H. *Oncogene* 2013, 32: 1164-1172.

[83] Kawamura K, Qi F, Meng Q, et al. Nucleolar protein nucleolin functions in replication stress-induced DNA damage responses. *J Radiat Res* 2019, 60: 281-288.

[84] Zhong Q, Hu Z, Li Q, et al. Cyclin D1 silencing impairs DNA double strand break repair, sensitizes BRCA1 wildtype ovarian cancer cells to olaparib. *Gynecol Oncol* 2019, 152: 157-165.

[85] Wan Q, Shen Y, Zhao H, et al. Impaired DNA double-strand breaks repair by kinesin family member 4A inhibition renders human H1299 non-small-cell lung cancer cells sensitive to cisplatin. *J Cell Physiol* 2019, 234: 10360-10371.

[86] Ishida T, Takizawa Y, Kainuma T, et al. DIDS, a chemical compound that inhibits RAD51-mediated homologous pairing and strand exchange. *Nucleic Acids Res* 2009, 37: 3367-3376.

[87] Kelso AA, Goodson SD, Chavan S, et al. Characterization of the recombination activities of the Entamoeba histolytica Rad51 recombinase. *Mol Biochem Parasitol* 2016, 210: 71-84.

[88] Lamont KR, Hasham MG, Donghia NM, et al. Attenuating homologous recombination stimulates an AID-induced antileukemic effect. *J Exp Med* 2013, 210: 1021-1033.

[89] Wilson JJ, Chow KH, Labrie NJ, et al. Enhancing the efficacy of glycolytic blockade in cancer cells via RAD51 inhibition. *Cancer Biol Ther* 2019, 20: 169-182.

[90] Li Y, He Y, Luo Y. Crystal structure of an archaeal Rad51 homologue in complex with a metatungstate inhibitor. *Biochemistry* 2009, 48: 6805-6810.

[91] Huang F, Motlekar NA, Burgwin CM, et al. Identification of specific inhibitors of human RAD51 recombinase using high-throughput screening. *ACS Chem Biol* 2011, 6: 628-635.

[92] Huang F, Mazina OM, Zentner IJ, et al. Inhibition of homologous recombination in human cells by targeting RAD51 recombinase. *J Med Chem* 2012, 55: 3011-3020.

[93] Huang F, Mazin AV. A small molecule inhibitor of human RAD51 potentiates breast cancer cell killing by therapeutic agents in mouse xenografts. *PloS One* 2014, 9: e100993.

[94] Budke B, Logan HL, Kalin JH, et al. RI-1: a chemical inhibitor of RAD51 that disrupts homologous recombination in human cells. *Nucleic Acids Res* 2012, 40: 7347-7357.

[95] Zhu J, Zhou L, Wu G, et al. A novel small molecule RAD51 inactivator overcomes imatinib-resistance in chronic myeloid leukaemia. *EMBO Mol Med* 2013, 5: 353-365.

[96] Normand A, Riviere E, Renodon-Corniere A. Identification and characterization of human Rad51 inhibitors by screening of an existing drug library. *Biochem Pharmacol* 2014, 91: 293-300.

[97] Chaudhuri AR, Callen E, Ding X, et al. Erratum: replication fork stability confers chemoresistance in BRCA-deficient cells. *Nature* 2016, 539: 456.

[98] Li X, Heyer WD. RAD54 controls access to the invading 3'-OH end after RAD51-mediated DNA strand invasion in homologous recombination in Saccharomyces cerevisiae. *Nucleic Acids Res* 2009, 37: 638-646.

[99] Lee RH, Slate DL, Moretti R, et al. Marine sponge polyketide inhibitors of protein tyrosine kinase. *Biochem Biophys Res Commun* 1992, 184: 765-772.

[100] Takaku M, Kainuma T, Ishida-Takaku T, et al. Halenaquinone, a chemical compound that specifically inhibits the secondary DNA binding of RAD51. *Genes Cell* 2011, 16: 427-436.

[101] Lv W, Budke B, Pawlowski M, et al. Development of small molecules that specifically inhibit the D-loop activity of RAD51. *J Med Chem* 2016, 59: 4511-4525.

[102] Choudhury A, Zhao H, Jalali F, et al. Targeting homologous recombination using imatinib results in enhanced tumor cell chemosensitivity and radiosensitivity. *Mol Cancer Ther* 2009, 8: 203-213.

[103] Zhao H, Luoto KR, Meng AX, et al. The receptor tyrosine kinase inhibitor amuvatinib (MP470) sensitizes tumor cells to radio- and chemo-therapies in part by inhibiting homologous recombination. *Radiother Oncol* 2011, 101: 59-65.

[104] Wang X, Gu Y, Liu H, et al. Icotinib hydrochloride enhances chemo- and radiosensitivity by inhibiting EGFR signaling and attenuating RAD51 expression and function in Hela S3 cells. *Onco Targets Ther* 2018, 11: 1245-1258.

[105] Ko JC, Ciou SC, Cheng CM, et al. Involvement of Rad51 in cytotoxicity induced by epidermal growth factor receptor inhibitor (gefitinib, IressaR) and chemotherapeutic agents in human lung cancer cells. *Carcinogenesis* 2008, 29: 1448-1458.

[106] Mihaila RG. From a better understanding of the mechanisms of action of histone deacetylases inhibitors to the progress of the treatment of malignant lymphomas and plasma cell myeloma. *Recent Patents Anticancer Drug Discov* 2017, 12: 283-295.

[107] Camphausen K, Scott T, Sproull M, et al. Enhancement of xenograft tumor radiosensitivity by the histone deacetylase inhibitor MS-275 and correlation with histone hyperacetylation. *Clin Cancer Res* 2004, 10: 6066-6071.

[108] Xie C, Drenberg C, Edwards H, et al. Panobinostat enhances cytarabine and daunorubicin sensitivities in AML cells through suppressing the expression of BRCA1, CHK1, and Rad51. *PloS One* 2013, 8: e79106.

[109] Adimoolam S, Sirisawad M, Chen J, et al. HDAC inhibitor PCI-24781 decreases RAD51 expression and inhibits homologous recombination. *Proc Natl Sci Acad USA* 2007, 104: 19482-19487.

[110] Majera D, Skrott Z, Bouchal J. Targeting genotoxic and proteotoxic stress-response pathways in human prostate cancer by clinically available PARP inhibitors, vorinostat and disulfiram. *Prostate* 2019, 79: 352-362.

[111] Gerelchuluun A, Maeda J, Manabe E, et al. Histone deacetylase inhibitor induced radiation sensitization effects on human cancer cells after photon and hadron radiation exposure. *Int J Mol Sci* 2018, 19: e496.

[112] Fenton M, Rathbone J, Reilly J, et al. Thioridazine for schizophrenia. *Cochrane Database Syst Rev* 2007, (3): Cd001944.

[113] Mao M, Yu T, Hu J, et al. Dopamine D2 receptor blocker thioridazine induces cell death in human uterine cervical carcinoma cell line SiHa. *J Obstet Gynaecol Res* 2015, 41: 1240-1245.

[114] Yong M, Yu T, Tian S, et al. DR2 blocker thioridazine: a promising drug for ovarian cancer therapy. *Oncol Lett* 2017, 14: 8171-8177.

[115] Brozovic A, Ambriovic-Ristov A, Osmak M. The relationship between cisplatin-induced reactive oxygen species, glutathione, and BCL-2 and resistance to cisplatin. *Crit Rev Toxicol* 2010, 40: 347-359.

[116] Li P, Yang X, Cheng Y, et al. MicroRNA-218 increases the sensitivity of bladder cancer to cisplatin by targeting Glut1. *Cell Physiol Biochem* 2017, 41: 921-932.

[117] Pantazaki AA, Lialiaris TS. A combined biochemical and cytogenetic study of thioridazine-induced damage to nucleic acids. *Mutagenesis* 1999, 14: 243-248.

[118] Spengler G, Csonka A, Molnar J, et al. The anticancer activity of the old neuroleptic phenothiazine-type drug thioridazine. *Anticancer Res* 2016, 36: 5701-5706.

[119] Shtam TA, Kovalev RA, Varfolomeeva EY, et al. Exosomes are natural carriers of exogenous siRNA to human cells in vitro. *Cell Commun Signal* 2013, 11: 88.

[120] Yu D, Zhang Y, Lu H, et al. Silver nanoparticles coupled to antiEGFR antibodies sensitize nasopharyngeal carcinoma cells to irradiation. *Mol Med Rep* 2017, 16: 9005-9010.

[121] Meena R, Kumar S, Kumar R, et al. PLGA-CTAB curcumin nanoparticles: fabrication, characterization and molecular basis of anticancer activity in triple negative breast cancer cell lines (MDA-MB-231 cells). *Biomed Pharmacother* 2017, 94: 944-954.

[122] Shetake NG, Kumar A, Pandey BN. Iron-oxide nanoparticles target intracellular HSP90 to induce tumor radio-sensitization. *Biochim Biophys Acta* 2019, 1863: 857-869.

In: Horizons in Cancer Research. Volume 73 ISBN: 978-1-53616-273-8
Editor: Hiroto S. Watanabe

Chapter 4

Multiple Myeloma: An Overview, Clinical Updates and Advances in Management

Haroon Majeed*, MBBS, MRCS, MSc, FEBOT, FRCS
Consultant Trauma & Orthopaedic Surgeon
Manchester University Foundation NHS Trust, Manchester, UK

Abstract

Multiple myeloma (MM) is an incurable malignant tumor of plasma cells of the bone marrow and is the most common primary neoplasm arising in bone. It causes approximately 1% of cancer-related deaths and is the 2nd commonest hematological malignancy in the western world. The median age at diagnosis is 69 years and it is an infrequent diagnosis before the age of 40 years.

Although the etiology of MM is not well-understood, it is thought to arise as a result of multiple genetic mutations of plasma cells and the immunoglobulins they produce. Some studies also suggest an association

* Corresponding Author's Email: haroon.majeed@nhs.net.

with occupational and environmental risk factors. Abnormalities of chromosome 13 are also detected in approximately 50% patients with MM.

Pathological fractures occur in approximately 40% patients. Bone disease also causes bone pain, spinal cord compression, diffuse osteoporosis and hypercalcemia, compromising mortality, morbidity and quality of life. Anemia, renal dysfunction and hypercalcemia are common metabolic complications and can range from mild to life-threatening. Immunosuppression, due to the disease itself and its treatment, can lead to frequent infections. Diagnosis depends on detection of M-proteins in plasma or urine, bone marrow biopsy, and end organ or bone damage.

Although MM remains incurable, improvements in treatment have had favorable impact on survival rates. Typical treatment combines alkylating chemotherapy drugs (Melaphan, Doxorubicin or Cyclophosphamide), a steroid (Dexamethazone or Prednisolone) and an immunomodulatory agent (Thalidomide, Lenalidomide or Bortezomib), depending on age and co-morbidities of the patients. Bisphosphonates are recommended for use in all symptomatic patients, of which Zoledronate and Pamidronate have proven efficacy. Radiotherapy is used to control pain and palliative treatment of focal lesions of disseminated disease.

Surgery has a supportive effect on long-term survival rates and quality of life in myeloma patients. Surgery is considered palliative in the majority of cases and surgical risks must be weighed against life expectancy and quality of life to justify surgical intervention. Stem cell transplantation combined with chemotherapy can be considered the standard of care in patients up to 65 years. Prognosis is highly variable, with overall estimated 35% survival at 5-years and 17% at 10-years with newer treatments.

Keywords: multiple myeloma, plasmacytoma, pathological fractures

1. Introduction

Multiple Myeloma (MM) is a malignant proliferation of neoplastic plasma cells of B-cell lineage within the bone marrow, leading to increased production of plasma paraprotein and immunoglobulin (Angtuaco et al. 2004). Myeloma is the second most common hematological malignancy and predominantly involves marrow-containing bones (vertebrae, pelvis and femur), however the lesions can occur in any bone as well as may involve lymph nodes and the skin (Harousseau, Shaughnessy, and Richardson 2004).

It is characterized by clonal expansion of malignant plasma cells resulting in end-organ damage, including lytic bone lesions, anemia, renal failure, or hypercalcemia (Mahindra et al. 2012). The first well-documented case of MM was reported in 1844 by Samuel Solly (Solly 1844). Although the disease remains incurable, the advances in treatment and supportive care have resulted in significant improvement in survival rates and associated morbidity over the past 20 years (Pozzi et al. 2013, Pulte et al. 2015).

2. EPIDEMIOLOGY

Geographically, the incidence of MM is reported to be the highest in Australia, Europe and North America (Becker 2011). MM is considered a disease of the elderly, which is reflected by the fact that the majority of cases are diagnosed in patients between the ages of 65 and 74 years (median age 69 years) (Howlader 2016). Approximately 35% to 40% of patients with MM are reported to be older than 75 years of age (Blade, Kyle, and Greipp 1996b). Less than 2% of patients diagnosed with MM are younger than 40 years of age and the incidence in patients younger than 30 years is extremely rare (Blade, Kyle, and Greipp 1996a). MM represents approximately 1.8% of all new cancer cases in the United States and accounted for just over 30,000 new cases in 2017 (Siegel, Miller, and Jemal 2017). The annual incidence has been reported to be 70 to 80 per million in the United Kingdom and it accounts for 2% of all the new cancer cases (Cancer Statistics UK 2015). The incidence of MM grows markedly with increasing age. Considering the worldwide population, elderly individuals older than 80 years are expected to increase from 3 million (current) to 6 million by 2030 indicating a proportionate increase in the number of patients with MM and this predicted fact necessitates appropriate strategies for its management (Gay and Larocca 2018).

3. Pathogenesis

Multiple myeloma arises as a result of multiple genetic mutations of plasma cells and the immunoglobulins they produce (Fonseca et al. 2004). Some studies have established an association with occupational and environmental risk factors (asbestos, farming, petroleum and ionizing radiation) (Eriksson and Karlsson 1992). There is also a suggestion of hereditary cause (Lynch et al. 2008). However, the evidence behind environmental and hereditary association is contradictory with the currently available research.

MM may arise *de novo* or from the pre-malignant condition 'monoclonal gammopathy of undetermined significance' (MGUS). The transitional events from MGUS to myeloma are not well-understood, however it is believed that it involves translocations of genes encoding both heavy-chains (IgH) and light-chains (IgL) (Fonseca et al. 2004). MGUS and smouldering multiple myeloma are asymptomatic forms of the disease (Eslick and Talaulikar 2013). In approximately 50% of patients chromosome 13 abnormalities are also detected and are considered to have a worse prognosis (Harousseau, Shaughnessy, and Richardson 2004). Mutation of tumor suppressor genes (ras, p53) is considered to be an important factor as well, however the prognostic significance of these is unclear (Fonseca et al. 2004). There is an up-regulation and over-expression of oncogenes and interferon regulatory factors leading to an increased cell survival and proliferation rate (Fonseca et al. 2004, Harousseau, Shaughnessy, and Richardson 2004).

Extensive research has been conducted to elucidate the different types of genetic aberrations in MM and their contributions to the disease establishment, progression, patient stratification and treatment (Manier et al. 2017). Based on the primary chromosomal alterations detected by karyotyping, MM can be divided into two major categories; the hyperdiploid and non-hyperdiploid MM (Avet-Loiseau et al. 2007, Fonseca et al. 2009). The hyperdiploid group is characterized by trisomies of odd-numbered chromosomes and has a favorable prognosis, while the non-hyperdiploid group is well known to harbor primary translocations involving the immunoglobulin heavy chain loci (IgH) and is associated with a poor prognosis (Alzrigat, Parraga, and Jernberg-Wiklund 2018).

In addition to secondary translocations and genetic aberrations, emerging data also suggest that epigenetic changes such as aberrant DNA methylation and histone modification profiles, and abnormal micro-RNA (miRNA) expression should be considered as important factors in contributing to the pathogenesis of MM (Popovic et al. 2014, Walker et al. 2011, Agarwal et al. 2016, Abdi, Qiu, and Chang 2014).

Multiple myeloma has several effects on the bone including focal osteolytic lesions, osteopenia, and elevated bone turnover. Myeloma cells induce the release of osteoclast activating factors Interleukin (IL-6, IL-1), tumor necrosis factor-b (TNF-b) and parathyroid hormone-related peptide (PTHrP), which consequently increase the cell surface expression of receptor activator of nuclear factor-kB (RANKL) on osteoblasts and stromal cells (Angtuaco et al. 2004, Sonmez et al. 2008). RANKL binds to RANK receptors on osteoclast precursors and triggers their differentiation into mature osteoclasts (Angtuaco et al. 2004). The uninhibited osteoclast activity releases cytokines from the bone matrix, which stimulates plasma cell proliferation and this vicious cycle continues to result in bone resorption, which in turn stimulates the myeloma cells leading to bone loss (Tricot 2000).

As large number of myeloma cells proliferate rapidly in the bone marrow, they begin to suffer from relative hypoxia, which results in release of angiogenic cytokines (vascular endothelial growth factor and fibroblast growth factor), which in turn stimulates angiogenesis (Andersen et al. 2005, Vacca and Ribatti 2006). This process triggers a vascular phase of proliferation of plasma cells leading to production of more cytokines and the disease process continues to accelerate (Fonseca et al. 2009).

4. Staging

The International Staging System (ISS) is used for staging multiple myeloma (Greipp et al. 2005). It is based on serum albumin and β-2 microglobulin (Table 1). The International Myeloma Working Group (IMWG) revised the ISS to enable better stratification of newly diagnosed myeloma patients (Table 2) (Palumbo et al. 2015). It was developed using 4000 patients, one-third of which were over 65 years of age and it now includes the detection of chromosomal abnormalities by interphase fluorescent in situ hybridization (iFISH) and the measurement of serum lactate dehydrogenase (LDH), which, when combined with the previous ISS, provides a powerful prognostic power compared with each individual parameter (Palumbo et al. 2015).

Table 1. International Staging System for Multiple Myeloma (Greipp et al. 2005)

Stage	Criteria	Median Survival (Months)
I	Serum β-2 microglobulin <3.5 mg/L and serum albumin >3.5g/dl	62
II	Neither I or III	45
III	Serum b-2 microglobulin >3.5 mg/l	29

Table 2. Revised International Staging System (Palumbo et al. 2015)

Prognostic Factor	
ISS stage	
I	Serum β_2-microglobulin < 3.5 mg/L, serum albumin ≥ 3.5 g/dL
II	Not ISS stage I or III
III	Serum β_2-microglobulin ≥ 5.5 mg/L
CA by iFISH	
High risk	Presence of del(17p) and/or translocation t(4;14) and/or translocation t(14;16)
Standard risk	No high-risk CA
LDH	
Normal	Serum LDH < the upper limit of normal
High	Serum LDH > the upper limit of normal
A new model for risk stratification for MM	
R-ISS stage	
I	ISS stage I and standard-risk CA by iFISH and normal LDH
II	Not R-ISS stage I or III
III	ISS stage III and either high-risk CA by iFISH or high LDH

Until a few years ago, MM patients were commonly defined as 'frail' if older than 75 years of age. During the recent years, different scores and indices have been developed that include a more complete geriatric assessment (Extermann et al. 2005). Geriatric assessment is an objective frailty predictor, which categorizes somatic, functional and psychological domains and is commonly used by geriatricians and oncologists in the decision-making process. In 2015, the International Myeloma Working Group (IMWG) developed a frailty score to determine the frailty status of patients and the feasibility of different treatment options (Fonseca et al. 2009). Based on a pooled-data of 869 newly diagnosed elderly patients enrolled in 3 prospective trials, an additive scoring system was developed to detect and define frailty based on age, Charlson Comorbidity Index (CCI), Activities of Daily Living (ADL) and Instrumental Activities of Daily Living (IADL) (Palumbo et al. 2015). Three groups were identified on the basis of this analysis: fit (score = 0, 39%); intermediate (score = 1, 31%), and frail patients (score ≥ 2, 30%).

Myeloma Comorbidity Index (MCI) is another useful tool to identify the geriatric risk profile of MM patients and carries a prognostic value for assessing functional decline and overall survival (Gay and Larocca 2018). Recently, renal and lung function, performance status impairment, frailty and age were combined in a weighted revised Myeloma Comorbidity Index (MCI), allowing for the identification of fit (Index ≤3), intermediate (Index 4–6) and frail patients (>6); indicating median overall survival rates of 10.1, 4.4 and 1.2 years, respectively (Engelhardt et al. 2017).

5. Assessment and Diagnosis

The International Myeloma Working Group (IMWG) has provided updated criteria for the diagnosis of multiple myeloma (Rajkumar et al. 2014), which includes:

a. Clonal bone marrow plasma cells greater than 10% or biopsy-proven bony or extramedullary plasmacytoma and any one or more of the following myeloma-defining events:
b. Evidence of end-organ damage
    i. Hypercalcemia
    ii. Renal insufficiency
    iii. Anemia
    iv. Bone lesions
c. Any one or more of the following biomarkers of malignancy:
    i. Clonal bone marrow plasma cell percentage of 60% or greater
    ii. Involved: uninvolved serum free light chain ratio of 100 or greater
    iii. Greater than 1 focal lesions on magnetic resonance imaging studies greater than 5 mm

The criteria described by International Myeloma Working Group for the diagnosis of asymptomatic and symptomatic myeloma is presented in Table 3 (Fonseca et al. 2009).

Table 3. Diagnostic Criteria for Multiple Myeloma

Monoclonal gammopathy of uncertain significance (MGUS)	Smouldering myeloma (SM)	Multiple myeloma (MM)
Serum monoclonal protein <30g/L	Serum monoclonal protein ≥30g/L	Monoclonal protein in serum and/or urine
Bone marrow clonal plasma cells <10%	Bone marrow monoclonal plasma cells ≥10%	Bone marrow clonal plasma cells or biopsy proven plasmacytoma
No evidence of other B cell lymphoproliferative disorders	No myeloma-related organ or tissue impairment	Myeloma-related organ or tissue impairment

a. Biochemical Markers

Evaluating a patient with suspected multiple myeloma involves establishing the evidence of a monoclonal paraprotein with serum electrophoresis (EPG) and immunofixation together with serum free-light-chain analysis (FLC) (Eslick and Talaulikar 2013). The combination of these three tests is considered to have a diagnostic sensitivity of 97–98% (Kyle and Rajkumar 2009). The remaining 2-3% of patients may have true non-secretory disease that is not detectable by any of these methods (Rajkumar 2013). Serum EPG analysis establishes the presence of a monoclonal band, while immunofixation further increases the diagnostic sensitivity and determines the precise nature of the paraproteins (IgA, IgG, IgM) (Eslick and Talaulikar 2013).

In addition, full blood count (FBC) and blood film, electrolytes including urea and creatinine, calcium, magnesium and phosphate analysis are mandatory to detect evidence of end-organ damage. For prognostic purposes, serum β2-microglobulin and albumin should also be assessed along with serum LDH levels. A referral to a hematologist should be made in order to obtain a bone marrow aspirate and trephine, immunehisto-chemistry, flow cytometry, and to guide further management (Fonseca et al. 2009).

b. Radiological Assessment

Plain Radiographs

As myeloma is primarily a disease of bone marrow, it can occur anywhere in the skeleton; therefore, a wide skeletal coverage is mandatory. Lytic lesions on conventional plain radiographs are typically circular punched-out lesions, without reconstruction, clearly visible on the cranial vault, the iliac bone or on the long bones (femur and humerus) (Touzeau and Moreau 2013). Vertebral compression is commonly seen and may be the first presenting symptom in a few cases. Once myeloma is diagnosed, a complete radiological assessment is necessary, which traditionally consist of plain radiographs of the skull, whole spine, pelvis, rib cage and long bones (humerus and femur only) (Touzeau and Moreau 2013). Approximately 80% of patients have obvious bone lesions, mainly affecting the spine (65%), ribs (45%) skull (40%), shoulder (40%), pelvis (30%) and the long bones (25%) (Touzeau and Moreau 2013). It is unusual to find lesions of the elbows or knees or further distally. Plain radiographs offer limited sensitivity because up to 50% of bone demineralization can occur before the lesions become evident on radiographs (Messiou and Kaiser 2018). It is important to keep in mind that up to 20% lesions are not visible on plain radiographs due to relatively poor sensitivity (Touzeau and Moreau 2013).

Computed Tomography (CT)

Whole-body CT can be used as a more sensitive alternative and has been reported to change of management plan in 18% to 61% of the patients compared with skeletal surveys (Kropil et al. 2008, Hillengass et al. 2017). CT has the advantages over conventional radiology as it is quicker relative to multiple standard radiographs, evaluates several lesions without having to reposition the patient keeping in view the painful lesions, is more effective for estimating a risk of fracture or instability, and can also pick up extra-medullary lesions (Touzeau and Moreau 2013). However, despite the use of low-dose radiation and improved sensitivity, the efficacy of CT remains inherently limited to primarily imaging the secondary effects of myeloma on cortical bone rather than bone marrow itself (Messiou and Kaiser 2018).

Magnetic Resonance Imaging (MRI)

Whole-body MR imaging is recognized as the gold-standard for the diagnosis of bone involvement in myeloma and in some countries it is recommended as the first-line imaging in patients with suspected diagnosis of myeloma (Messiou and Kaiser 2018). MRI provides greater sensitivity, extremely precise localization of the lesions in axial skeleton, discrimination between normal and invaded bone marrow, good visualization of extra-medullary lesions and other associated conditions (cardiac amyloidosis) (Walker et al. 2007). It is also valuable in evaluation of the therapeutic response of treatment. The MRI appearance and a number of lesions more than or equal to 7 are considered major prognostic factors and more important than the cytogenetics (Touzeau and Moreau 2013).

Positron Emission Tomography (PET)

PET scan in myeloma is still not fully validated. However, emerging data suggest that the use and efficacy of PET scan will grow considerably in the coming years. It provides a highly attractive combination of anatomic and functional information albeit at radiation doses 4 to 5 times higher than those used in low-dose CT alone (Touzeau and Moreau 2013). Some studies have shown that the number of lesions found at the time of diagnosis is an important prognostic factor. PET scan can also be valuable in assessing the therapeutic response (Zamagni et al. 2011).

c. Bone Marrow Biopsy

The definitive diagnosis of MM requires analysis of a bone marrow biopsy and is recommended in all cases (Bird et al. 2011). An appropriate sample is considered to be 20 mm that yields superior results to traditional bone marrow aspirate. The sample is assessed by flow cytometry or immunohistochemistry to detect antigen and the results are analyzed against The International Myeloma Working Group diagnostic criteria as discussed earlier.

6. Clinical Presentation

Myeloma Bone Disease

Approximately 80–90% of myeloma patients suffer from osteolytic lesions during the course of disease affecting axial and appendicular skeleton. Bone disease in myeloma may result in severe bone pain (70-80%), pathological fractures (50-60%), hypercalcemia (15%), spinal cord compression (2-3%) and diffuse osteoporosis, all of which contribute to further compromise in mobility, independence and quality of life (Sonmez et al. 2008, Bird et al. 2011, Hameed et al. 2014). Pathological fractures commonly occur in the thoracic and lumbar spine (Figure 1) but may also occur in ribs, skull (Figure 2), pelvis, femur (Figure 3) and humerus (Figure 4) (Angtuaco et al. 2004). Vertebral compression fractures significantly increase the risk of spinal cord compression and an estimated 32% increase in mortality (Sonmez et al. 2008).

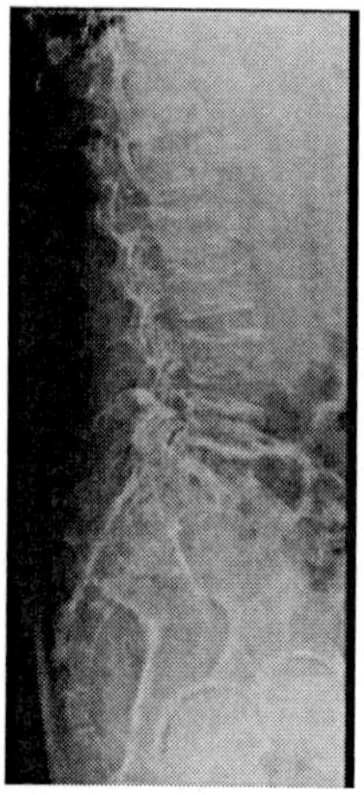

Figure 1. Plain radiograph lateral view showing multiple pathological fractures in lumbar spine in a patient with myeloma. (Case courtesy of Dr Hani Salam, Radiopaedia.org, rID: 8508. No formal permission required to reproduce the image as per Radiopedia.org guidance.)

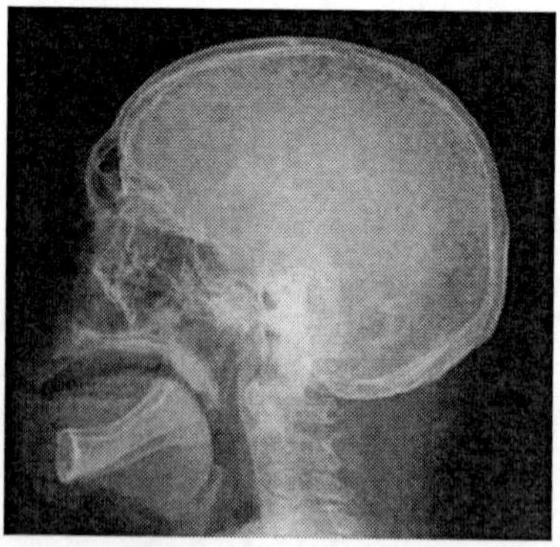

Figure 2. Plain radiograph lateral view with typical punched out lesion of myeloma in skull. (Case courtesy of Dr Mohammad Taghi Niknejad, Radiopaedia.org, rID: 61511. No formal permission required to reproduce the image as per Radiopedia.org guidance.)

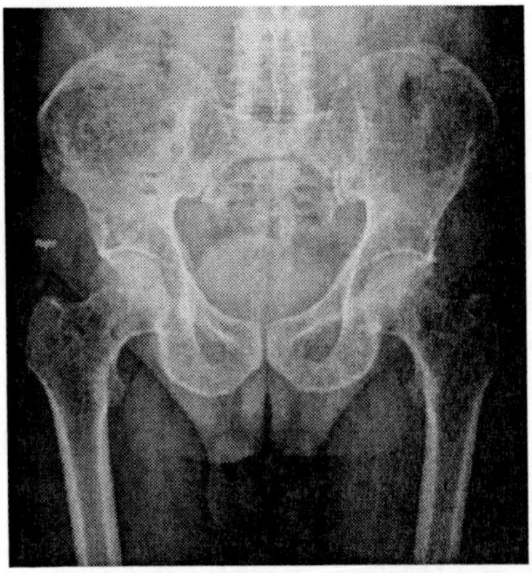

Figure 3. Plain radiograph anteroposterior view of pelvis and both proximal femori showing multiple osteolytic lesions in a patient with MM. (Case courtesy of Dr Mohammad Taghi Niknejad, Radiopaedia.org, rID: 61511. No formal permission required to reproduce the image as per Radiopedia.org guidance.)

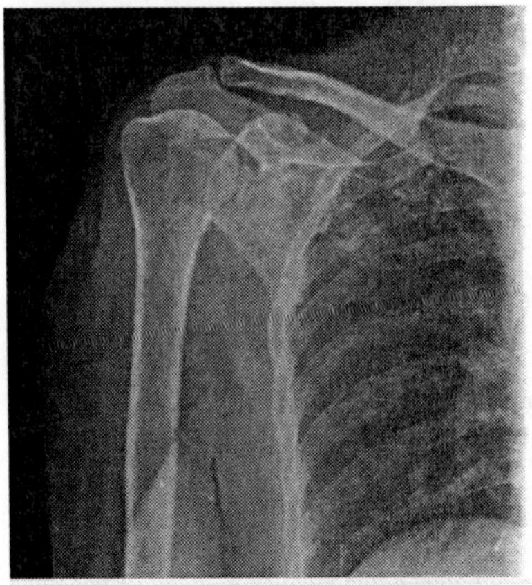

Figure 4. Plain anteroposterior radiograph of right humerus with multiple small lytic lesions. (Case courtesy of Dr Saikat Sarkar, Radiopaedia.org, rID: 54702. No formal permission required to reproduce the image as per Radiopedia.org guidance.)

Hypercalcemia

Hypercalcemia is the most common metabolic complication of myeloma due to increased osteoclastic activity and is seen in one third of the patients (Oyajobi 2007). Depending on serum calcium levels, the clinical presentation of hypercalcemia may vary; either completely asymptomatic or may present with symptoms of confusion, depression, polyuria, polydipsia, constipation, nausea and in cases of higher levels, may lead to coma (hypercalcemic crisis) (Tricot 2000).

Renal Dystrophy

Renal dysfunction in myeloma occurs secondary to amyloidosis, light chain cast nephropathy and the nephrotoxic effects of chemotherapeutic agents used for treatment (Faiman et al. 2011). In patients with symptomatic myeloma renal dysfunction is common and may progress to end-stage renal failure necessitating dialysis during the course of the disease (Harousseau, Shaughnessy, and Richardson 2004). Chronic renal disease induces renal osteodystrophy and secondary hyperparathyroidism worsening the potential for skeletal complication in patients with MM (Faiman et al. 2011).

Immunosuppression

Immunosuppression in MM results from a combination of factors that include immunological dysfunction, immunosuppressive therapeutic agents and medical comorbidities. The use of corticosteroids, chemotherapy, immune-modulating agents and stem cell transplant cause iatrogenic suppression of the immune system (Nucci and Anaissie 2009). Patients with MM are prone to develop recurrent infections, of which, pneumonia and septicemia are most common and may progress on to neutropenic sepsis (Pratt, Goodyear, and Moss 2007).

Anemia

More than two-thirds of the patients with MM present with anemia, which further adds on to the morbidity and the quality of life in these patients (Mittelman 2003). It occurs due to a combination of factors including the chronicity of the disease process, suppression of erythropoietin by cytokines and renal impairment, and chemotherapy-induced myelosuppression (Barlogie et al. 2004).

7. Management of Multiple Myeloma

Multiple myeloma remains an incurable disease and long-term remissions are seen in few patients. Management of MM and its associated bone disease requires a multidisciplinary approach including antimyeloma treatment and the use of other supportive modalities like Bisphosphonates, radiotherapy, pain management, vertebroplasy, kyphoplasty (Figure 5) and other surgical interventions (Hameed et al. 2014). The choice of appropriate treatment is challenging and many factors need to be carefully considered (Gay and Larocca 2018). The optimal strategy should balance efficacy and toxicity of the treatment used, especially in frail patients making the afore-mentioned geriatric assessment a valuable tool to assess elderly patients and modulate treatment objectives based on their frailty status (Extermann et al. 2005). The dose adjustment and efficacy of the treatment is dependent on the age and comorbidities of the patient. In addition, frailty and compromised organ function also make the patients more vulnerable to side effects, poor compliance and early treatment discontinuation (Gay and Larocca 2018). A large meta-analysis (1435 elderly patients enrolled in 4 randomized trials) demonstrated that the risk of death was higher in patients aged 75 years or above and patients with renal failure, infections or cardiac/gastrointestinal adverse events during treatment (Bringhen et al. 2013).

The goals of treatment vary in different patients based on their medical fitness (Gay and Larocca 2018):

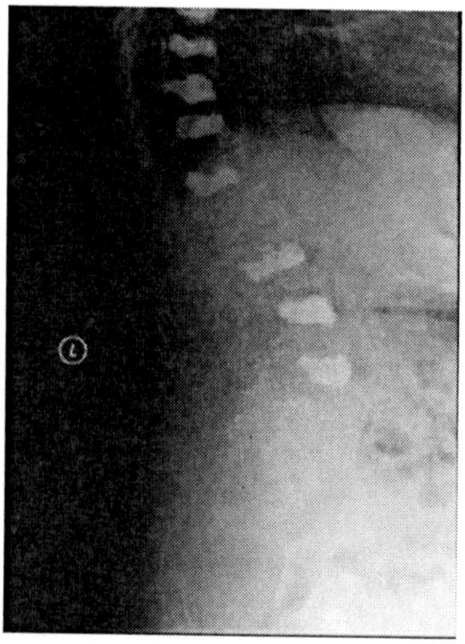

Figure 5. Plain radiograph lateral view of a patient with MM treated with cement augmentation for multiple vertebral compression fracture in thoraco-lumbar spine. (Case courtesy of Radswiki, Radiopaedia.org, rID: 11643. No formal permission required to reproduce the image as per Radiopedia.org guidance.)

a. The goal of therapy for fit patients is to achieve a complete remission and improve survival.
b. For intermediate fit or frail patients, for whom comorbidities and treatment toxicities hamper efficacy of full-dose therapy, the main objective of treatment is to improve and preserve the quality of life for as long as possible.

Pain Management

Pain in MM occurs due to the disease process and bone resorption. It is the primary complaint of most of the patients with MM (70-80%) (Sonmez et al. 2008). In some cases it can also occur due to nerve root compression and as a side effect of some medications (Thalidomide or Bortezomib) (Hameed et al. 2014). In patients with mild pain, simple analgesics are recommended (Paracetamol). Patients with moderate to severe pain may benefit from opioid medications (Tramadol, Oxycodone, Fentanyl patches and Morphine). Bisphosphonates are also helpful in pain control (Snowden et al. 2011). In cases where pain does not settle with pharmacological treatment, other modalities like radiotherapy, vertebroplasty/kyphoplasty and other surgical interventions may be indicated (Siemionow and Lieberman 2008, Majeed, Bommireddy, and Klezl 2014).

Bisphosphonates

Bisphosphonate therapy (BPT) is considered as a standard treatment for myeloma bone disease. Their main function is inhibition of osteoclast maturation and formation, enhancement of osteoclast apoptosis, and reduction of their adherence to bone by inhibition of farnesyl pyrophosphate synthase (Dunford et al. 2001). Pamidronate and Zoledronic Acid are widely used nitrogen-containing Bisphosphonates in intravenous form as the oral forms are considered less effective in MM. They are recommended in symptomatic myeloma, with or without the evidence of bone disease (Snowden et al. 2011). Dose adjustment is required for Zoledronic Acid in cases of renal impairment; however, Pamidronate can be used in patients with severe renal impairment by extending the duration of the infusion (Snowden et al. 2011). Another adverse effect of BPT is osteonecrosis of the mandible (1 to 10%) that warrants regular dental follow-up (Durie 2007).

IMWG suggested discontinuing BPT after one year in patients in complete remission or in good partial remission and no active bone disease (Fonseca et al. 2009). Patients with ongoing bone disease should Have BPT for up to 2 years, after which it can be stopped if there is no suggestion of active bone disease. In cases with persistent bone disease, further use of BPT is at the discretion of treating physician with a preferable choice of Pamidronate.

Immunosuppressive Agents

Typical treatment for MM combines alkylating chemotherapy drugs (Melaphan, Doxorubicin or Cyclophosphamide), a steroid (Dexamethazone or Prednisolone) and an immunomodulatory agent (Thalidomide or Lenalidomide) or more recently proteasome inhibitors (Bortezomib) (Barlogie et al. 2004). These drugs are well-known for causing their myelosuppressive and immunosuppressive side effects as well as associated with peripheral neuropathies, cardiomyopathies and thromboembolism (Barlogie et al. 2004). Multiple trials have demonstrated superior survival rates with the use of Melphalan-Prednisone-Thalidomide (MPT) or Bortezomib-Melphalan-Prednisone (VMP) over Melphalan and Prednisone (MP) alone (Gavriatopoulou et al. 2018).

Radiotherapy

Radiotherapy is used to control pain (success rate up to 90%) and palliative treatment of focal lesions in cases of wide-spread disease. Radiotherapy may also promote healing of pathological fractures once surgically stabilized however; it does not influence prognosis or survival in these patients (Bird et al. 2011). Other indications include spinal cord compression, soft tissue lesions and control of local neurological symptoms. Major risk of radiotherapy is permanent bone marrow damage, which can affect stem cell harvest in future (Leigh et al. 1993).

Surgical Intervention

Surgery has a supportive role in the management of MM. Although considered palliative in the majority of cases, however has shown to improve quality of life and overall survival in some patients (Utzschneider et al. 2011). Surgery aims to decompress or stabilize vertebral fractures with instability and/or neurological deficit, stabilize pathological fractures (including impending fractures) and to manage the pain (Hameed et al. 2014, Angtuaco et al. 2004). Cement augmentation (vertebroplasty or kyphoplasty) is also used in these patients. Vertebroplasty is a minimally invasive procedure under fluoroscopic guidance during which bone cement is injected into the collapsed vertebral body for stabilization or pain relief. Kyphoplasty is the addition of an inflatable balloon that is placed into the vertebral body to expand it and followed by injection of bone cement (Majeed, Bommireddy, and Klezl 2014). Both these procedures are associated with potential leakage of cement into the spinal canal resulting in nerve irritation, cord compression and embolization of the cement (Garland, Gishen, and Rahemtulla 2011). However, these are considered effective and safe in reduction of pain and improvement of mobility in patients with vertebral compression fractures. The decision of undertaking surgery in patients with MM is not straightforward and requires a multidisciplinary approach together with hematologist and oncologist.

Newer Treatments

A series of recently published pivotal phase III trials has established the role of second-generation protease inhibitors (Carfilzomib, Ixazomib, Elotuzumab and Daratumumab) in relapsed or refractory MM (Wildes 2017).

Carfilzomib is an intravenously-administered drug which irreversibly inhibits the chymotrypsin-like proteasome, causing inhibition of proliferation and apoptosis (Kuhn et al. 2007). It was approved for relapsed MM in the United States in 2012 and by the European Commission in 2015.

Ixazomib is an orally-administered therapy, which reversibly inhibits the chymotrypsin-like activity of the proteasome, inducing apoptosis (Chauhan et al. 2011). In the United States, it was approved by FDA in combination with Lenalidomide for relapsed myeloma in 2015. The European Commission granted conditional authorization in the same combination in 2016.

Elotuzumab is a monoclonal antibody that targets the cell surface molecule CS1/SLAMF7 (signaling lymphocyte activation marker F7), inducing antibody dependent cellular cytotoxicity (ADCC) (Hsi et al. 2008). It was approved in combination with Lenalidomide for relapsed MM in the US in 2015 and by the European Commission in 2016.

Daratumumab is a human monoclonal antibody directed against the CD38 expressed on MM cells. It induces ADCC and complement-dependent cytotoxicity (de Weers et al. 2011). It was approved in the US in 2015 and in Europe in 2016 as a single agent for MM patients who have received both a proteasome inhibitor and an immunomodulatory agent.

Marizomib and *Oprozomib* are still in the first phase of clinical development. Marizomib is an oral, non-peptidic, irreversible protease inhibitor, isolated from the marine actinomycete salinispora tropica (Hungria et al. 2019). It binds irreversibly to the three catalytic subunits of the 20S proteasome. Oprozomib is an oral, irreversible protease inhibitor derived from Carfilzomib, which demonstrates Carfilzomib-like potency in cytotoxicity assays (Hungria et al. 2019). A number of trials are ongoing to evaluate the efficacy and toxicity profiles of these newer agents and therapy combinations.

Stem Cell Transplant

Stem cell transplant (SCT) is commonly used to treat multiple myeloma in patients under the age of 65 years; however it is also feasible in selected patients older than 65 years who have good performance status and no severe comorbidities (Manapuram and Hashmi 2018). High dose drug treatment is used to reduce the number of myeloma cells prior to the transplant (Kyle and Rajkumar 2009). Stem cell transplant can be autologous or allogeneic. Over the past two decades, the proportion of adults older than 70 years undergoing autologous SCT has increased more than five-fold, from less than 1% to 5% (Wildes, Rosko, and Tuchman 2014). Some studies have reported superior results of a combined high dose therapy with SCT over chemotherapy alone in patients between 50 and 70 years of age (Palumbo et al. 2010), while some others have reported conflicting results in patients between 65 and 70 years of age (Facon et al. 2007).

8. Survival and Prognosis

Multiple myeloma is an incurable condition, however as with most cancers, survival rates are improving, which are attributable to earlier diagnosis, better detection, effective and widespread use of high-dose chemotherapy and autologous stem cell transplantation over the last 2 decades (Renshaw et al. 2010). According to the SEER (Surveillance, Epidemiology, and End Results) data for multiple myeloma published by the National Cancer Institute the average life expectancy has gone up from 4 years to 5.5 years (SEER 2018). It is difficult to make survival comparisons between different countries due to different methodologies and criteria used for including patients in these analyses.

In the United States (US), the survival rates have improved by an impressive 300 percent; from a median survival of 2.5 years after diagnosis in 1997 to more than 10 years in 2012. Between 2000 and 2009, there has been a reported 73 percent increase in the number of myeloma survivors in the US (Altekruse, Kosary, and Krapch 2010).

In England and Wales, one-year age-standardized net survival for myeloma has increased from 37% during 1971-1972 to 78% during 2010-2011 (survival difference of 41 percentage points) in men and from 38% to 75% over the same time period (a difference of 37 percentage points) in women (Cancer Research UK).

Five-year survival for myeloma decreases with increasing age. Across the European countries, five-year survival rates range from 23.1% to 46.7% (Woods et al. 2010). Myeloma survival continues to fall beyond five years after diagnosis (Woods et al. 2010).

Ten-year survival has increased by a lesser amount than one- and five-year survival since the early 1970s. Ten-year age-standardized net survival in men has increased from 7% during 1971-1972 to a predicted survival of 37% during 2010-2011 in England and Wales (survival difference of 29 percentage points) and in women, this has increased from 6% to 28% over the same time period (survival difference of 23 percentage points) (Cancer Research UK). Overall, a third of patients diagnosed with myeloma today are predicted to survive their disease for at least ten years.

In myeloma patients who sustain a long bone fracture, mean survival has been shown to fall from 57 months to 18 months, however following surgical fixation of the fracture the mean survival improves again to 47 months (Sonmez et al. 2008). Myeloma survivors may experience long-term consequences of their disease itself and side effects of the treatment used. These primarily include peripheral neuropathy, venous thrombo-embolism, recurrent infections and gastrointestinal problems (Bird et al. 2011).

In summary, there have been major recent advancements in the understanding and management of multiple myeloma. Establishing the diagnosis rests on identifying a monoclonal paraprotein in the serum and confirming the presence of myeloma-related organ or tissue injury, followed by a multidisciplinary approach with hematologist and oncologist to establish further management. It is important to assess each patient's clinical situation and fitness for therapy to allow treatment to be provided at an appropriate intensity. The availability of new combination therapies including novel agents and enhanced safety of autologous stem cell transplant has increased the treatment options for elderly patients with multiple myeloma and improved the survival rates over the past 2 decades.

REFERENCES

Abdi, J., L. Qiu, and H. Chang. 2014. "Micro-RNAs, New performers in multiple myeloma bone marrow microenvironment." *Biomark Res* 2:10. doi: 10.1186/2050-7771-2-10.

Agarwal, P., M. Alzrigat, A. A. Parraga, S. Enroth, U. Singh, J. Ungerstedt, A. Osterborg, P. J. Brown, A. Ma, J. Jin, K. Nilsson, F. Oberg, A. Kalushkova, and H. Jernberg-Wiklund. 2016. "Genome-wide profiling of histone H3 lysine 27 and lysine 4 trimethylation in multiple myeloma reveals the importance of Polycomb gene targeting and highlights EZH2 as a potential therapeutic target." *Oncotarget* 7 (6):6809-23. doi: 10.18632/oncotarget.6843.

Altekruse, S. F., C. l. Kosary, and M. Krapch. 2010. "*SEER Cancer Statistics Review, 1975–2007.*" Bethesda, MD: National Cancer Institute; 2010.

Alzrigat, M., A. A. Parraga, and H. Jernberg-Wiklund. 2018. "Epigenetics in multiple myeloma: From mechanisms to therapy." *Semin Cancer Biol* 51:101-115. doi: 10.1016/j.semcancer.2017.09.007.

Andersen, N. F., T. Standal, J. L. Nielsen, L. Heickendorff, M. Borset, F. B. Sorensen, and N. Abildgaard. 2005. "Syndecan-1 and angiogenic cytokines in multiple myeloma: correlation with bone marrow angiogenesis and survival." *Br J Haematol* 128 (2):210-7. doi: 10.1111/j.1365-2141.2004.05299.x.

Angtuaco, E. J., A. B. Fassas, R. Walker, R. Sethi, and B. Barlogie. 2004. "Multiple myeloma: clinical review and diagnostic imaging." *Radiology* 231 (1):11-23. doi: 10.1148/radiol.2311020452.

Avet-Loiseau, H., M. Attal, P. Moreau, C. Charbonnel, F. Garban, C. Hulin, S. Leyvraz, M. Michallet, I. Yakoub-Agha, L. Garderet, G. Marit, L. Michaux, L. Voillat, M. Renaud, B. Grosbois, G. Guillerm, L. Benboubker, M. Monconduit, C. Thieblemont, P. Casassus, D. Caillot, A. M. Stoppa, J. J. Sotto, M. Wetterwald, C. Dumontet, J. G. Fuzibet, I. Azais, V. Dorvaux, M. Zandecki, R. Bataille, S. Minvielle, J. L. Harousseau, T. Facon, and C. Mathiot. 2007. "Genetic abnormalities and survival in multiple myeloma: the experience of the Intergroupe Francophone du Myelome." *Blood* 109 (8):3489-95. doi: 10.1182/blood-2006-08-040410.

Barlogie, B., J. Shaughnessy, G. Tricot, J. Jacobson, M. Zangari, E. Anaissie, R. Walker, and J. Crowley. 2004. "Treatment of multiple myeloma." *Blood* 103 (1):20-32. doi: 10.1182/blood-2003-04-1045.

Becker, N. 2011. "Epidemiology of multiple myeloma." *Recent Results Cancer Res* 183:25-35. doi: 10.1007/978-3-540-85772-3_2.

Bird, J. M., R. G. Owen, S. D'Sa, J. A. Snowden, G. Pratt, J. Ashcroft, K. Yong, G. Cook, S. Feyler, F. Davies, G. Morgan, J. Cavenagh, E. Low, J. Behrens, Haematology Haemato-oncology Task Force of British Committee for Standards in, and U. K. Myeloma Forum. 2011.

"Guidelines for the diagnosis and management of multiple myeloma 2011." *Br J Haematol* 154 (1):32-75. doi: 10.1111/j.1365-2141.2011.08573.x.

Blade, J., R. A. Kyle, and P. R. Greipp. 1996a. "Multiple myeloma in patients younger than 30 years. Report of 10 cases and review of the literature." *Arch Intern Med* 156 (13):1463-8.

Blade, J., R. A. Kyle, and P. R. Greipp. 1996b. "Presenting features and prognosis in 72 patients with multiple myeloma who were younger than 40 years." *Br J Haematol* 93 (2):345-51.

Bringhen, S., M. V. Mateos, S. Zweegman, A. Larocca, A. P. Falcone, A. Oriol, D. Rossi, M. Cavalli, P. Wijermans, R. Ria, M. Offidani, J. J. Lahuerta, A. M. Liberati, R. Mina, V. Callea, M. Schaafsma, C. Cerrato, R. Marasca, L. Franceschini, A. Evangelista, A. I. Teruel, B. van der Holt, V. Montefusco, G. Ciccone, M. Boccadoro, J. San Miguel, P. Sonneveld, and A. Palumbo. 2013. "Age and organ damage correlate with poor survival in myeloma patients: meta-analysis of 1435 individual patient data from 4 randomized trials." *Haematologica* 98 (6):980-7. doi: 10.3324/haematol.2012.075051.

Cancer Research UK. "https://www.cancerresearchuk.org/health-professional/cancer-statistics/statistics-by-cancer-type/myeloma/survival#ref-2."

Cancer Statistics UK 2015. "No authors listed. Cancer registration statistics, England Statistical bulletins, https://www.ons.gov.uk/peoplepopulationandcommunity/healthandsocialcare/conditionsanddiseases/bulletins/cancerregistrationstatisticsengland/previousReleases."

Chauhan, D., Z. Tian, B. Zhou, D. Kuhn, R. Orlowski, N. Raje, P. Richardson, and K. C. Anderson. 2011. "In vitro and in vivo selective antitumor activity of a novel orally bioavailable proteasome inhibitor MLN9708 against multiple myeloma cells." *Clin Cancer Res* 17 (16):5311-21. doi: 10.1158/1078-0432.CCR-11-0476.

de Weers, M., Y. T. Tai, M. S. van der Veer, J. M. Bakker, T. Vink, D. C. Jacobs, L. A. Oomen, M. Peipp, T. Valerius, J. W. Slootstra, T. Mutis, W. K. Bleeker, K. C. Anderson, H. M. Lokhorst, J. G. van de Winkel, and P. W. Parren. 2011. "Daratumumab, a novel therapeutic human

CD38 monoclonal antibody, induces killing of multiple myeloma and other hematological tumors." *J Immunol* 186 (3):1840-8. doi: 10.4049/jimmunol.1003032.

Dunford, J. E., K. Thompson, F. P. Coxon, S. P. Luckman, F. M. Hahn, C. D. Poulter, F. H. Ebetino, and M. J. Rogers. 2001. "Structure-activity relationships for inhibition of farnesyl diphosphate synthase in vitro and inhibition of bone resorption in vivo by nitrogen-containing bisphosphonates." *J Pharmacol Exp Ther* 296 (2):235-42.

Durie, B. G. 2007. "Use of bisphosphonates in multiple myeloma: IMWG response to Mayo Clinic consensus statement." *Mayo Clin Proc* 82 (4):516-7; author reply 517-8. doi: 10.4065/82.4.516.

Engelhardt, M., A. S. Domm, S. M. Dold, G. Ihorst, H. Reinhardt, A. Zober, S. Hieke, C. Baayen, S. J. Muller, H. Einsele, P. Sonneveld, O. Landgren, M. Schumacher, and R. Wasch. 2017. "A concise revised Myeloma Comorbidity Index as a valid prognostic instrument in a large cohort of 801 multiple myeloma patients." *Haematologica* 102 (5):910-921. doi: 10.3324/haematol.2016.162693.

Eriksson, M., and M. Karlsson. 1992. "Occupational and other environmental factors and multiple myeloma: a population based case-control study." *Br J Ind Med* 49 (2):95-103.

Eslick, R., and D. Talaulikar. 2013. "Multiple myeloma: from diagnosis to treatment." *Aust Fam Physician* 42 (10):684-8.

Extermann, M., M. Aapro, R. Bernabei, H. J. Cohen, J. P. Droz, S. Lichtman, V. Mor, S. Monfardini, L. Repetto, L. Sorbye, E. Topinkova, and C. G. A. of the International Society of Geriatric Oncology Task Force on. 2005. "Use of comprehensive geriatric assessment in older cancer patients: recommendations from the task force on CGA of the International Society of Geriatric Oncology (SIOG)." *Crit Rev Oncol Hematol* 55 (3):241-52. doi: 10.1016/j. critrevonc.2005.06.003.

Facon, T., J. Y. Mary, C. Hulin, L. Benboubker, M. Attal, B. Pegourie, M. Renaud, J. L. Harousseau, G. Guillerm, C. Chaleteix, M. Dib, L. Voillat, H. Maisonneuve, J. Troncy, V. Dorvaux, M. Monconduit, C. Martin, P. Casassus, J. Jaubert, H. Jardel, C. Doyen, B. Kolb, B. Anglaret, B. Grosbois, I. Yakoub-Agha, C. Mathiot, H. Avet-Loiseau, and Myelome

Intergroupe Francophone du. 2007. "Melphalan and prednisone plus thalidomide versus melphalan and prednisone alone or reduced-intensity autologous stem cell transplantation in elderly patients with multiple myeloma (IFM 99-06): a randomised trial." *Lancet* 370 (9594):1209-18. doi: 10.1016/S0140-6736(07)61537-2.

Faiman, B. M., P. Mangan, J. Spong, J. D. Tariman, and Board The International Myeloma Foundation Nurse Leadership. 2011. "Renal complications in multiple myeloma and related disorders: survivorship care plan of the International Myeloma Foundation Nurse Leadership Board." *Clin J Oncol Nurs* 15 Suppl:66-76. doi: 10.1188/11.CJON.S1.66-76.

Fonseca, R., B. Barlogie, R. Bataille, C. Bastard, P. L. Bergsagel, M. Chesi, F. E. Davies, J. Drach, P. R. Greipp, I. R. Kirsch, W. M. Kuehl, J. M. Hernandez, S. Minvielle, L. M. Pilarski, J. D. Shaughnessy, Jr., A. K. Stewart, and H. Avet-Loiseau. 2004. "Genetics and cytogenetics of multiple myeloma: a workshop report." *Cancer Res* 64 (4):1546-58.

Fonseca, R., P. L. Bergsagel, J. Drach, J. Shaughnessy, N. Gutierrez, A. K. Stewart, G. Morgan, B. Van Ness, M. Chesi, S. Minvielle, A. Neri, B. Barlogie, W. M. Kuehl, P. Liebisch, F. Davies, S. Chen-Kiang, B. G. Durie, R. Carrasco, O. Sezer, T. Reiman, L. Pilarski, H. Avet-Loiseau, and Group International Myeloma Working. 2009. "International Myeloma Working Group molecular classification of multiple myeloma: spotlight review." *Leukemia* 23 (12):2210-21. doi: 10.1038/leu.2009.174.

Garland, P., P. Gishen, and A. Rahemtulla. 2011. "Percutaneous vertebroplasty to treat painful myelomatous vertebral deposits-long-term efficacy outcomes." *Ann Hematol* 90 (1):95-100. doi: 10.1007/s00277-010-1021-2.

Gavriatopoulou, M., D. Fotiou, I. Ntanasis-Stathopoulos, E. Kastritis, E. Terpos, and M. A. Dimopoulos. 2018. "How I treat elderly patients with plasma cell dyscrasias." *Aging (Albany NY)* 10 (12):4248-4268. doi: 10.18632/aging.101707.

Gay, F., and A. Larocca. 2018. "Special problems in the management of elderly patients with multiple myeloma." *Eur J Intern Med* 58:64-69. doi: 10.1016/j.ejim.2018.05.027.

Greipp, P. R., J. San Miguel, B. G. Durie, J. J. Crowley, B. Barlogie, J. Blade, M. Boccadoro, J. A. Child, H. Avet-Loiseau, R. A. Kyle, J. J. Lahuerta, H. Ludwig, G. Morgan, R. Powles, K. Shimizu, C. Shustik, P. Sonneveld, P. Tosi, I. Turesson, and J. Westin. 2005. "International staging system for multiple myeloma." *J Clin Oncol* 23 (15):3412-20. doi: 10.1200/JCO.2005.04.242.

Hameed, A., J. J. Brady, P. Dowling, M. Clynes, and P. O'Gorman. 2014. "Bone disease in multiple myeloma: pathophysiology and management." *Cancer Growth Metastasis* 7:33-42. doi: 10.4137/ CGM.S16817.

Harousseau, J. L., J. Shaughnessy, Jr., and P. Richardson. 2004. "Multiple myeloma." *Hematology Am Soc Hematol Educ Program*:237-56. doi: 10.1182/asheducation-2004.1.237.

Hillengass, J., L. A. Moulopoulos, S. Delorme, V. Koutoulidis, J. Mosebach, T. Hielscher, M. Drake, S. V. Rajkumar, B. Oestergaard, N. Abildgaard, M. Hinge, T. Plesner, Y. Suehara, K. Matsue, N. Withofs, J. Caers, A. Waage, H. Goldschmidt, M. A. Dimopoulos, S. Lentzsch, B. Durie, and E. Terpos. 2017. "Whole-body computed tomography versus conventional skeletal survey in patients with multiple myeloma: a study of the International Myeloma Working Group." *Blood Cancer J* 7 (8):e599. doi: 10.1038/bcj.2017.78.

Howlader, N; Noone, AM; Krapcho, M. 2016. "*SEER Cancer Statistics Review, 1975–2013, based on November 2015 SEER data submission, posted to the SEER web site.*"

Hsi, E. D., R. Steinle, B. Balasa, S. Szmania, A. Draksharapu, B. P. Shum, M. Huseni, D. Powers, A. Nanisetti, Y. Zhang, A. G. Rice, A. van Abbema, M. Wong, G. Liu, F. Zhan, M. Dillon, S. Chen, S. Rhodes, F. Fuh, N. Tsurushita, S. Kumar, V. Vexler, J. D. Shaughnessy, Jr., B. Barlogie, F. van Rhee, M. Hussein, D. E. Afar, and M. B. Williams. 2008. "CS1, a potential new therapeutic antibody target for the treatment of multiple myeloma." *Clin Cancer Res* 14 (9):2775-84. doi: 10.1158/1078-0432.CCR-07-4246.

Hungria, V. T. M., E. Q. Crusoe, R. I. Bittencourt, A. Maiolino, R. J. P. Magalhaes, J. D. N. Sobrinho, J. V. Pinto, R. C. Fortes, E. S. Moreira, and P. Y. Tanaka. 2019. "New proteasome inhibitors in the treatment of multiple myeloma." *Hematol Transfus Cell Ther* 41 (1):76-83. doi: 10.1016/j.htct.2018.07.003.

Kropil, P., R. Fenk, L. B. Fritz, D. Blondin, G. Kobbe, U. Modder, and M. Cohnen. 2008. "Comparison of whole-body 64-slice multidetector computed tomography and conventional radiography in staging of multiple myeloma." *Eur Radiol* 18 (1):51-8. doi: 10.1007/s00330-007-0738-3.

Kuhn, D. J., Q. Chen, P. M. Voorhees, J. S. Strader, K. D. Shenk, C. M. Sun, S. D. Demo, M. K. Bennett, F. W. van Leeuwen, A. A. Chanan-Khan, and R. Z. Orlowski. 2007. "Potent activity of carfilzomib, a novel, irreversible inhibitor of the ubiquitin-proteasome pathway, against preclinical models of multiple myeloma." *Blood* 110 (9):3281-90. doi: 10.1182/blood-2007-01-065888.

Kyle, R. A., and S. V. Rajkumar. 2009. "Criteria for diagnosis, staging, risk stratification and response assessment of multiple myeloma." *Leukemia* 23 (1):3-9. doi: 10.1038/leu.2008.291.

Leigh, B. R., T. A. Kurtts, C. F. Mack, M. B. Matzner, and D. S. Shimm. 1993. "Radiation therapy for the palliation of multiple myeloma." *Int J Radiat Oncol Biol Phys* 25 (5):801-4.

Lynch, H. T., K. Ferrara, B. Barlogie, E. A. Coleman, J. F. Lynch, D. Weisenburger, W. Sanger, P. Watson, H. Nipper, V. Witt, and S. Thome. 2008. "Familial myeloma." *N Engl J Med* 359 (2):152-7. doi: 10.1056/NEJMoa0708704.

Mahindra, A., J. Laubach, N. Raje, N. Munshi, P. G. Richardson, and K. Anderson. 2012. "Latest advances and current challenges in the treatment of multiple myeloma." *Nat Rev Clin Oncol* 9 (3):135-43. doi: 10.1038/nrclinonc.2012.15.

Majeed, H., R. Bommireddy, and Z. Klezl. 2014. "Cement augmentation for vertebral fractures in patients with multiple myeloma." *Acta Orthop Belg* 80 (4):551-7.

Manapuram, S., and H. Hashmi. 2018. "Treatment of Multiple Myeloma in Elderly Patients: A Review of Literature and Practice Guidelines." *Cureus* 10 (12):e3669. doi: 10.7759/cureus.3669.

Manier, S., K. Z. Salem, J. Park, D. A. Landau, G. Getz, and I. M. Ghobrial. 2017. "Genomic complexity of multiple myeloma and its clinical implications." *Nat Rev Clin Oncol* 14 (2):100-113. doi: 10.1038/nrclinonc.2016.122.

Messiou, C., and M. Kaiser. 2018. "Whole-Body Imaging in Multiple Myeloma." *Magn Reson Imaging Clin N Am* 26 (4):509-525. doi: 10.1016/j.mric.2018.06.006.

Mittelman, M. 2003. "The implications of anemia in multiple myeloma." *Clin Lymphoma* 4 Suppl 1:S23-9.

Nucci, M., and E. Anaissie. 2009. "Infections in patients with multiple myeloma." *Semin Hematol* 46 (3):277-88. doi: 10.1053/j.seminhematol.2009.03.006.

Oyajobi, B. O. 2007. "Multiple myeloma/hypercalcemia." *Arthritis Res Ther* 9 Suppl 1:S4. doi: 10.1186/ar2168.

Palumbo, A., H. Avet-Loiseau, S. Oliva, H. M. Lokhorst, H. Goldschmidt, L. Rosinol, P. Richardson, S. Caltagirone, J. J. Lahuerta, T. Facon, S. Bringhen, F. Gay, M. Attal, R. Passera, A. Spencer, M. Offidani, S. Kumar, P. Musto, S. Lonial, M. T. Petrucci, R. Z. Orlowski, E. Zamagni, G. Morgan, M. A. Dimopoulos, B. G. Durie, K. C. Anderson, P. Sonneveld, J. San Miguel, M. Cavo, S. V. Rajkumar, and P. Moreau. 2015. "Revised International Staging System for Multiple Myeloma: A Report From International Myeloma Working Group." *J Clin Oncol* 33 (26):2863-9. doi: 10.1200/JCO.2015.61.2267.

Palumbo, A., S. Bringhen, B. Bruno, A. P. Falcone, A. M. Liberati, M. Grasso, R. Ria, F. Pisani, C. Cangialosi, T. Caravita, A. Levi, G. Meloni, A. Nozza, P. Pregno, A. Gabbas, V. Callea, M. Rizzo, L. Annino, V. De Stefano, P. Musto, I. Baldi, F. Cavallo, M. T. Petrucci, M. Massaia, and M. Boccadoro. 2010. "Melphalan 200 mg/m(2) versus melphalan 100 mg/m(2) in newly diagnosed myeloma patients: a prospective, multicenter phase 3 study." *Blood* 115 (10):1873-9. doi: 10.1182/blood-2009-09-241737.

Popovic, R., E. Martinez-Garcia, E. G. Giannopoulou, Q. Zhang, Q. Zhang, T. Ezponda, M. Y. Shah, Y. Zheng, C. M. Will, E. C. Small, Y. Hua, M. Bulic, Y. Jiang, M. Carrara, R. A. Calogero, W. L. Kath, N. L. Kelleher, J. P. Wang, O. Elemento, and J. D. Licht. 2014. "Histone methyltransferase MMSET/NSD2 alters EZH2 binding and reprograms the myeloma epigenome through global and focal changes in H3K36 and H3K27 methylation." *PLoS Genet* 10 (9):e1004566. doi: 10.1371/journal.pgen.1004566.

Pozzi, S., L. Marcheselli, A. Bari, E. V. Liardo, R. Marcheselli, S. Luminari, M. Quaresima, C. Cirilli, P. Ferri, M. Federico, and S. Sacchi. 2013. "Survival of multiple myeloma patients in the era of novel therapies confirms the improvement in patients younger than 75 years: a population-based analysis." *Br J Haematol* 163 (1):40-6. doi: 10.1111/bjh.12465.

Pratt, G., O. Goodyear, and P. Moss. 2007. "Immunodeficiency and immunotherapy in multiple myeloma." *Br J Haematol* 138 (5):563-79. doi: 10.1111/j.1365-2141.2007.06705.x.

Pulte, D., L. Jansen, F. A. Castro, K. Emrich, A. Katalinic, B. Holleczek, H. Brenner, and Gekid Cancer Survival Working Group. 2015. "Trends in survival of multiple myeloma patients in Germany and the United States in the first decade of the 21st century." *Br J Haematol* 171 (2):189-196. doi: 10.1111/bjh.13537.

Rajkumar, S. V. 2013. "Multiple myeloma: 2013 update on diagnosis, risk-stratification, and management." *Am J Hematol* 88 (3):226-35. doi: 10.1002/ajh.23390.

Rajkumar, S. V., M. A. Dimopoulos, A. Palumbo, J. Blade, G. Merlini, M. V. Mateos, S. Kumar, J. Hillengass, E. Kastritis, P. Richardson, O. Landgren, B. Paiva, A. Dispenzieri, B. Weiss, X. LeLeu, S. Zweegman, S. Lonial, L. Rosinol, E. Zamagni, S. Jagannath, O. Sezer, S. Y. Kristinsson, J. Caers, S. Z. Usmani, J. J. Lahuerta, H. E. Johnsen, M. Beksac, M. Cavo, H. Goldschmidt, E. Terpos, R. A. Kyle, K. C.

Anderson, B. G. Durie, and J. F. Miguel. 2014. "International Myeloma Working Group updated criteria for the diagnosis of multiple myeloma." *Lancet Oncol* 15 (12):e538-48. doi: 10.1016/S1470-2045(14)70442-5.

Renshaw, C., N. Ketley, H. Moller, and E. A. Davies. 2010. "Trends in the incidence and survival of multiple myeloma in South East England 1985-2004." *BMC Cancer* 10:74. doi: 10.1186/1471-2407-10-74.

SEER 2018. "Surveillance, Epidemiology, and End Results (SEER) Program (www.seer.cancer.gov) Research Data (1973-2015), National Cancer Institute, DCCPS, Surveillance Research Program, released April 2018, based on the November 2017 submission.".

Siegel, R. L., K. D. Miller, and A. Jemal. 2017. "Cancer Statistics, 2017." *CA Cancer J Clin* 67 (1):7-30. doi: 10.3322/caac.21387.

Siemionow, K., and I. H. Lieberman. 2008. "Surgical approaches to metastatic spine disease." *Curr Opin Support Palliat Care* 2 (3):192-6. doi: 10.1097/SPC.0b013e32830c9060.

Snowden, J. S., J. C. Thompson, C. L. Stopford, A. M. Richardson, A. Gerhard, D. Neary, and D. M. Mann. 2011. "The clinical diagnosis of early-onset dementias: diagnostic accuracy and clinicopathological relationships." *Brain* 134 (Pt 9):2478-92. doi: 10.1093/brain/awr189.

Solly, S. 1844. "Remarks on the pathology of mollities ossium; with cases." *Med Chir Trans* 27:435-498 8.

Sonmez, M., T. Akagun, M. Topbas, U. Cobanoglu, B. Sonmez, M. Yilmaz, E. Ovali, and S. B. Omay. 2008. "Effect of pathologic fractures on survival in multiple myeloma patients: a case control study." *J Exp Clin Cancer Res* 27:11. doi: 10.1186/1756-9966-27-11.

Touzeau, C., and P. Moreau. 2013. "Multiple myeloma imaging." *Diagn Interv Imaging* 94 (2):190-2. doi: 10.1016/j.diii.2012.12.003.

Tricot, G. 2000. "New insights into role of microenvironment in multiple myeloma." *Lancet* 355 (9200):248-50. doi: 10.1016/S0140-6736(00)00019-2.

Utzschneider, S., H. Schmidt, P. Weber, G. P. Schmidt, V. Jansson, and H. R. Durr. 2011. "Surgical therapy of skeletal complications in multiple myeloma." *Int Orthop* 35 (8):1209-13. doi: 10.1007/s00264-010-1127-0.

Vacca, A., and D. Ribatti. 2006. "Bone marrow angiogenesis in multiple myeloma." *Leukemia* 20 (2):193-9. doi: 10.1038/sj.leu.2404067.

Walker, B. A., C. P. Wardell, L. Chiecchio, E. M. Smith, K. D. Boyd, A. Neri, F. E. Davies, F. M. Ross, and G. J. Morgan. 2011. "Aberrant global methylation patterns affect the molecular pathogenesis and prognosis of multiple myeloma." *Blood* 117 (2):553-62. doi: 10.1182/blood-2010-04-279539.

Walker, R., B. Barlogie, J. Haessler, G. Tricot, E. Anaissie, J. D. Shaughnessy, Jr., J. Epstein, R. van Hemert, E. Erdem, A. Hoering, J. Crowley, E. Ferris, K. Hollmig, F. van Rhee, M. Zangari, M. Pineda-Roman, A. Mohiuddin, S. Yaccoby, J. Sawyer, and E. J. Angtuaco. 2007. "Magnetic resonance imaging in multiple myeloma: diagnostic and clinical implications." *J Clin Oncol* 25 (9):1121-8. doi: 10.1200/JCO.2006.08.5803.

Wildes, T. M. 2017. "Emerging therapies for multiple myeloma: Application in older adults." *J Geriatr Oncol* 8 (6):413-416. doi: 10.1016/j.jgo.2017.07.006.

Wildes, T. M., A. Rosko, and S. A. Tuchman. 2014. "Multiple myeloma in the older adult: better prospects, more challenges." *J Clin Oncol* 32 (24):2531-40. doi: 10.1200/JCO.2014.55.1028.

Woods, L. M., B. Rachet, L. Shack, D. Catney, P. M. Walsh, N. Cooper, C. White, V. Mak, J. Steward, H. Comber, A. Gavin, D. Brewster, M. Quinn, M. P. Coleman, and U. K. Association of Cancer Registries. 2010. "Survival from twenty adult cancers in the UK and Republic of Ireland in the late twentieth century." *Health Stat Q* (46):5-24. doi: 10.1057/hsq.2010.9.

Zamagni, E., F. Patriarca, C. Nanni, B. Zannetti, E. Englaro, A. Pezzi, P. Tacchetti, S. Buttignol, G. Perrone, A. Brioli, L. Pantani, C. Terragna, F. Carobolante, M. Baccarani, R. Fanin, S. Fanti, and M. Cavo. 2011. "Prognostic relevance of 18-F FDG PET/CT in newly diagnosed multiple myeloma patients treated with up-front autologous transplantation." *Blood* 118 (23):5989-95. doi: 10.1182/blood-2011-06-361386.

Biographical Sketch

Haroon Majeed

Affiliation: Manchester University Foundation NHS Trust, Manchester, United Kingdom

Education: MBBS; MRCS; MSc; FEBOT; FRCS (Tr & Orth)

Business Address: Manchester Royal Infirmary, Oxford Road, Manchester, United Kingdom M13 9WL

Research and Professional Experience:

- Masters Degree in Trauma and Orthopedics
- Principle Investigator of Randomized Controlled Trials
- Leading role in multiple quality improvement projects
- Published 28 research articles including RCT, meta-analysis, systematic reviews, prospective studies, case series and book chapters
- Presented research work at 45 occasions internationally, nationally and regionally

Professional Appointments: Consultant Trauma and Orthopedic Surgeon, Manchester University Foundation NHS Trust

Honors: BOA National Fellowship, BOA Clinical Leaders Certification, Travelling Fellowship in Foot and Ankle Surgery (Germany)

Publications from the Last 3 Years:

- Silastic replacement of the first metatarsophalangeal joint; historical evolution, modern concepts and a systematic review of the literature. *EFORT Open Reviews*; 2019;4:77-84.

- Survivorship and long-term outcome of a consecutive series of 200 Scandinavian Total Ankle Replacement (STAR) implants. *Bone Joint J.* 2019;101-B:47–54.
- Effect on Hospital Length of Stay of Tourniquet Use During Internal Fixation of Ankle Fractures: Randomized Controlled Trial. *The Journal of Foot & Ankle Surgery* 58(1) Jan 2019, 114-118.
- Total ankle arthroplasty; What are the risks; A guide to surgical consent and review of the literature. *Bone Joint J* 2018;100-B:1352–8.
- Turf toe injury; Current concepts and an updated review of the literature. *Foot Ankle Clin N Am;* Epub ahead of print, Sep 2018.
- Minimally invasive reduction and percutaneous fixation versus open reduction and internal fixation for displaced intra-articular calcaneal fractures; a systematic review of literature. *EFORT Open Reviews;* Vol 3; July 18.
- Talar Process Fractures; an overview and update of literature. *EFORT Open Reviews;* 2018;3:85-92.
- Direct anterior approach versus posterior approach for total hip arthroplasty; short-term results of functional assessment in the early phase of recovery. *Orthopaedic Surgery and Traumatology* 1.6, 203-214.
- Massive Patellar Tendon Ossification: Excision and Simultaneous Total Knee Replacement. *Scientific Pages Orthop Surg* 2017, 1(1):17-19, Volume 1 | Issue 1.
- Effect of Cold Weather on the Symptoms of Arthritic Disease: A Review of the Literature. *Journal of General Practice,* Vol 4: Issue 5, Nov 2016.
- Which one is a valuable surrogate for predicting survival between Tomita and Tokuhashi scores in patients with spinal metastases? A meta-analysis for diagnostic test accuracy and individual participant data analysis; *J Neurooncol*, DOI 10.1007/s11060-015-1794-1, May 2015.

- Multiple intratendinous ossified deposits of the Achilles tendon; Case report of an unusual pattern of ossification. *Foot and Ankle Surgery;* Vol. 21, Issue 2, e33–e35.
- All inside meniscal repair surgery; factors affecting the outcome. *Journal of Orthopaedics and Traumatology*; DOI 10.1007/s10195-015-0342-2. Feb 2015.
- Failure of meniscal repair in association with late anterior cruciate ligament reconstruction. *Journal of Orthopaedics;* DOI:10.1016/j.jor.2015.01.031. Feb 2015.

In: Horizons in Cancer Research. Volume 73 ISBN: 978-1-53616-273-8
Editor: Hiroto S. Watanabe

Chapter 5

INFECTIOUS COMPLICATIONS IN MULTIPLE MYELOMA

Nina Kumar[1] and Lokesh Shahani[2,*], MD

[1]Rice University, Houston, TX, US

[2]Department of Psychiatry, UT Houston McGovern Health Center, Houston, TX, US

ABSTRACT

Multiple myeloma, a hematological malignancy characterized by the proliferation of malignant plasma cells within the bone marrow, is associated with reduced immunity. Multiple myeloma related immunodeficiency involves B-cell dysfunction and abnormalities of T-cells, dendritic cells, and NK-cells. The literature shows that patients with multiple myeloma display a low immune response to infections and vaccines, have a higher risk of infection, and most importantly, note that infectious diseases are the leading cause of death in these patients. Recent studies have reported an evolving range of infections in multiple myeloma, likely due to new therapies including stem cell therapies, novel agents, and monoclonal antibodies. This book chapter will briefly review the

* Corresponding Author's Email: Lokesh.R.Shahani@uth.tmc.edu.

prevalence and types of infectious complications that patients with multiple myeloma face as well as present and emerging therapeutic approaches.

Keywords: multiple myeloma, malignancy, infections, antibiotic prophylaxis

INTRODUCTION

Multiple myeloma is a clonal plasma cell malignancy that constitutes 1% of all cancers worldwide and 10-15% of hematological neoplasms, and is the third most commonly occurring disease of the blood after leukemia and non-Hodgkin lymphoma.[1] Risk factors for multiple myeloma include older age, exposure to ionizing radiation, benzene, herbicides, insecticides, and most relevant to this review, immunosuppression. [2]

Infections are a significant cause of morbidity and mortality in multiple myeloma patients given their immunosuppression. There are several reports in the literature that patients with multiple myeloma have impaired immune function, and the reasons for this are multi-fold. Some factors that explain the impaired immune function include hypogamma-globulinemia, impaired lymphocyte function, steroid-related immunosup-pression, neutropenia secondary to chemotherapy or marrow infiltration, and physical factors such as indwelling catheters, impaired mucosal integrity, and respiratory distress. [3] Some studies have shown that the incidence of infectious episodes in multiple myeloma occur from 0.80-2.22 per year, nearly 7-15 times greater than patients hospitalized for other causes. [4] One study found that bacterial and viral infections were seven times higher in patients with multiple myeloma compared to controls with bacterial infections such as pneumonia and septicemia and viral infections such as herpes zoster and influenza is significantly higher in multiple myeloma patients. [5] Studies have reported the main sites of infection to be the respiratory and urinary tracts, and several studies have explored the types of bacteria and viruses that cause infections in patients with multiple myeloma. [4]

One reason for the increasing incidence of infection in multiple myeloma are the several new and emerging therapies for multiple myeloma. Therapies include allogeneic transplant, vaccine therapy, immunomodulatory drugs, epigenetic approaches, adaptive T-cell therapy, and monoclonal antibodies. [5] Monoclonal antibodies in particular seem to be generating a certain amount of excitement with some monoclonal antibodies targeting multiple myeloma cell antigens, some targeting immune inhibitory molecules, and adoptive cellular therapy. Despite these new treatment's efficacy, it is important to recognize the immune-suppressive risks they hold and management options. Our review will briefly cover the prevalence and types of infectious complications seen in multiple myeloma patients as well as the effects of the new and emerging therapies mentioned above and management options for infections.

Basics of Multiple Myeloma

Multiple myeloma (MM) is the second most common hematologic malignancy after lymphoma, accounting for 1% of all cancers. [6, 8] It accounts for 17% of hematologic malignancies in the United States specifically, with the annual incidence in the United States approximately 4-5 per 100,000 individuals. [9, 10] A recent systematic analysis of the global burden of MM found age-standardized incidence and death rates to be highest in the North American, Australasian, and Western European populations and lowest in Asia, Oceania, and sub-Saharan Africa, in line with previous studies. [11] Regarding other demographic factors, MM is more common in African Americans compared to their white counterparts; the literature shows that not only is MM 2-3 times more common in blacks but also reveals a younger age of onset and higher MM-specific mortality rates in these patients. [12] MM generally affects older adults; the median age at diagnosis is currently 66 years of age, with only 10% and 2% of patients younger than 50 and 40 years respectively. [13, 14] One study examining demographic trends in MM patients from 1993 to 2010 examining the future demographics of MM states that from 2011 to 2034,

MM will primarily affect individuals aged 64-84 years with 3 of every 4 newly diagnosed MM patients in this age group (an increase from ~2 out of every 3 patients today) and the percentage of racial/ethnic minorities affected will increase regardless of gender (29% to 37% among men and 34% to 38% among women). [15] Men are more likely than women to be affected by MM; the American Cancer Society estimates in 2019 that of 32,110 new cases diagnosed in 2019, 18,130 will be in men and 13, 980 in women. [16] Multiple myeloma is a malignant proliferation of multifocal neoplastic plasma cells in the bone marrow in which malignant monoclonal B cells differentiate into plasma cells. [17] In myeloma bone disease, increased osteoclastogenesis with suppressed osteoblastic activity leads to bone lesions in the form of discrete lytic lesions, widespread osteopenia, or multiple lytic lesions affecting any part of the skeleton, though generally preferring the spine, skull, and long bones. [18] The end result is a number of organ dysfunctions and symptoms of bone pain or fractures, renal failure, susceptibility to infection, anemia, hypercalcemia, and occasionally clotting abnormalities, neurologic symptoms, and manifestations of hyperviscosity. [19]

MM begins as monoclonal gammopathy of undetermined significance (MGUS), progresses to smoldering (asymptomatic) myeloma, and finally becomes overt (symptomatic) myeloma with the normal equilibrium between osteoblastic and osteoclastic activity becoming skewed towards net bone loss as the disease progresses. [20] MGUS progresses to multiple myeloma with a probability that increases 1% every year. [21] The molecular pathophysiology explaining the change from normal plasma cells to malignant plasma cells is unclear, but involves dysregulation of the cyclin D proteins (cyclins D1, D2, and D3) through multiple mechanisms including translocations of cyclin D1 and D3 with the IgH gene, specific cyclin D gene amplifications, trisomies, and other cytogenetic events that are not yet characterized. [8] Essentially, MM cells directly stimulate osteoclast formation and induce cells in the microenvironment to produce factors that drive formation of osteoclasts, while also inducing cells in the microenvironment to increase production of osteoblastic suppressors. [22] Tumor and stromal cells interact via adhesion molecules and cytokine networks to promote tumor cell survival, drug resistance, angiogenesis, and disordered bone metabolism. [23] Myeloma cells themselves produce osteoclast-activating factors including receptor activator of NF-kB ligand (RANKL), macrophage inflammatory protein 1-alpha (MIP-1α), interleukin (IL)-3 and tumor necrosis factor-alpha (TNF-α), while also inducing marrow stromal cell production of growth factors that enhance osteoclast formation including RANKL, IL-6, TNF-α and that decrease production of osteoclast inhibitory factors. The factors produced by the marrow stromal cells and osteoclasts promote tumor growth through direct action on MM cells. [22] The process of bone destruction releases bone matrix-derived growth factors such as transforming growth factor-beta (TGFß), insulin-like growth factors (IGFs), fibroblast growth factors (FGFs), platelet-derived growth factor (PDGF), and bone morphogenic proteins (BMPs) that increase the growth of myeloma cells, further driving the osteolytic process. MM cells also induce other cells in the marrow microenvironment to increase production of osteoblastic suppressors such as sclerostin made by osteocytes, TNF-α, and growth factor independent 1 transcriptional repressor (GFI1) made by marrow stromal cells. MM cells also induce marrow stromal cells to produce factors that support the myeloma cells including IL-6, vascular cell adhesion protein 1 (VCAM1), VEGF, and IGF-1. Immunologically active compounds involved in these processes include TGF-*β*, IL-10, IL-6, VEGF, Fas ligand, Mucin-1 (Muc-1), cyclooxygenase-2 (COX-2) and related prostanoids, and matrix metalloproteinases (MMPs).**Error! Bookmark not defined.** [23] Myeloma cells produce excess TGF-*β* which suppresses T-cell responses against tumor cells via inhibition of IL-2 autocrine pathways in T cells and stimulation of T regulatory (Treg) cell proliferation; IL-10 is produced by myeloma cells and has an unclear effect on the immune system; Muc-1 skews the differentiation of dendritic cells, acts as a chemoattractant for immature dendritic cells, and may have a role in the direct apoptosis of T cells; VEGF inhibits T-cell development in mice, inhibits maturation of dendritic cells, augments proinflammatory T-cell differentiation, and promotes IL-6 production; and IL-6 blocks dendritic cell maturation and inhibits dendritic cell function. [23] MM cells also express proangiogenic genes aberrantly compared to normal cells—97% of MM samples express at least one angiogenic factor among the 6 most frequently expressed factors, including hepatocyte growth factor (HGF). [24] Stimulating MM cells with HGF is correlated with activating signaling pathways that are associated in regulation of cell proliferation and survival. The immune system plays an important role in the pathogenesis of MM, and its role also explains why those with MM are more susceptible to infections. Studies have found that the levels of B cells, NK cells, and CD4+ T cells are much lower compared to normal control as well as the immunoglobulin reduction (a clinical feature found in symptomatic MM). [25] The main dysregulated immunological components in MM include dendritic cells, Treg, Th17, and myeloid derived suppressor cells (MDSC). It is surmised that the combination of expansion of particular Treg cells (CD25+ Foxp3+), secretion of proangiogenic cytokines within the MM environment, enhanced tryptophan catabolism, expression of co-inhibitory receptors and other immune suppressive molecules, dendritic cell dysfunction, weak immunogenicity of MM-associated Id proteins, and maintenance of clonogenic MM precursors cause immune dysfunction in individuals with MM and lead to an increased risk of infection. [24] The pathology of MM is important and has prognostic significance with three different types of plasma cells recognized: mature, intermediate, and immature or plasmablastic cells. [27] The immature plasma cells are associated with worse prognosis and proliferation of the disease. Specific cytological features to be aware of that can indicate MM include nuclear pleomorphism (variations reported in the literature include cytoplasm invaginations in the nucleus, invaginations of the inner nuclear membrane, nuclear lobulation, multinuclearity, and Dutcher bodies), variations in cytoplasmic clearing (Russell bodies, mott cells, grape cells, signet-ring-like cells, flaming cells), and a high nucleo-cytoplasmic ratio. [27] These variations can be categorized into three prognostic grades based on the predominant plasma cell type: Marschalko or low grade (small cell), intermediate (cleaved, polymorphous, asynchronous), and high grade (blastic) with the latter grade seen in 10-15% of MM patients during their initial phase of disease and associated with poorer prognosis. [27]

There are two specific therapeutic categories for treatment of MM: proteasome inhibitors and immunomodulatory drugs, both with notable side effects that affect the immune system. The best known proteasome inhibitor is Bortezomib, which inhibits the activity of the 26S proteasome by blocking the degradation of IκBα, an inhibitory protein that is constitutively bound to cytosolic NF-κB, thereby inhibiting the nuclear translocation and activation of NF-κB. [26] Bortezomib also inhibits IL-6, induces apoptosis by activating caspase-8 and caspase-9 in drug-resistant MM cell lines, and downregulates the expression of adhesion molecules on MM cells and bone marrow stromal cells. [26] Given the various functions that bortezomib has, it should not be unsurprising that its immune-suppressive roles can have multiple negative effects on different immune cells including a decrease in CD4 T-cell count, lessened CD8 T-cell cytotoxicity *in* vitro, impaired antibody-mediated responses by enhanced B-cell apoptosis, and a host of negative effects pertaining to dendritic cells (including desensitized dendritic cells to immunostimulation by tumor necrosis factor-α (TNF-α), induction of apoptosis in dendritic cells, loss of antigen presentation, reduction of dendritic cell induced allogenic T-cell proliferation, and inhibition of the expression of dendritic cell maturation markers), all of which lead to increased infections in the patient. [27] The incidence rate of infection complications seen in bortezomib varies depending on the study: one study found a 13% incidence of varicella zoster virus (VZV) infection in newly diagnosed MM patients on bortezomib; another study found that 75% of patients treated with melphalan, prednisone, and bortezomib had at least 1 episode of infection during treatment; and another study found that the highest rate of infections was in the "bortezomib-based protocols" group with 50% infection, though this was thought to be because this protocol was used as salvage treatment for patients with severe cumulative malfunction of the immune system. [28, 29, 30] The other category contains thalidomide and its analogues (second generation includes lenalidomide and pomalidomide), which inhibit TNF-α production and angiogenesis by blocking the angiogenic growth factors, basic fibroblast growth factor, and VEGF, inhibit Tregs, trigger apoptosis by activating caspase-8 and caspase-9, inhibit production of proinflammatory cytokines such as IL-1, IL-6, IL-2, and TNF-α and inhibiting angiogenesis and enhance NK cell proliferation and activity against MM cells. [26, 31] Similar to bortezomib, use of thalidomide or its structural analogs is associated with significant toxicities such as neutropenia, myelosuppression, thrombocytopenia, and serious infections given its many function as an immunosuppressant in the treatment of MM. [32] One study showed that despite antibiotic prophylaxis, 38.5% of studied patients (out of 224) on thalidomide for MM developed infections with the majority developing pneumonia (59%). [33] However, other studies report that thalidomide is not significant myelotoxic and was not found to increase the risk of infection in newly diagnosed patients in multiple RCTs of dexamethasone versus dexamethasone plus thalidomide and melphalan plus prednisone versus melphalan plus prednisone with thalidomide. [34, 35]

Another viable treatment option for MM is stem cell transplantation. Hematopoietic stem cell transplant (HSCT) refers to the transplantation of hematopoietic cells originating in the bone marrow following cytotoxic and immunosuppressive therapy for treatment of malignant and benign diseases. [36] Autologous HSCT (ASCT) refers to the situation in which the donor and the recipient is the same person. In the two largest studies, ASCT showed a 12-month improvement in overall survival compared with nontransplant cohorts, though this was performed before the introduction of novel agents so may not be as current. [37] Another RCT comparing chemotherapy plus lenalidomide with ASCT versus lenalidomide-prednisone or lenalidomide alone in newly diagnosed MM patients revealed significantly prolonged progression-free survival in the transplant arm (60% versus 38% at 3 years). [37] Tandem (double) ASCT can be performed in which the patient receives a second ASCT after recovery from the first procedure; randomized trials have found significantly better event-free survival and overall survival in recipients of tandem versus single ASCT. [39] ASCT is recommended for patients with MM who are relatively young and do not have any serious co-existing illnesses; while a formal age limit is not imposed in the United States, transplantation is only considered in patients 64 years of age or younger in Europe. [38] Allogeneic transplantation is discouraged given the high morbidity related to graft versus host disease, and the fact that data from randomized trials regarding the benefit of allogeneic stem cell transplantation are conflicting. [39] The process of ASCT includes induction treatment (3-6 cycles of chemotherapy with dexamethasone or combined with thalidomide, bortezomib, or lenalidomide, stem-cell collection and high-dose chemotherapy, followed by infusion of the transplanted cells with the whole duration of treatment lasting 4-6 months. [38] The use of ASCT as a first-line therapy has been questioned given the presence of safer and more effective agents such as pomalidomide, and the fact that ASCT only prolongs progression-free survival and overall survival, but is not curative. [40] One study from 1998 to 2011 looking at in-hospital complications from transplant found the most common complications to be stomatitis (44.7%), anemia requiring transfusion (28.5%), febrile neutropenia (16.5%), and bacteremia (15.0%), and noted that despite increase in age and number of comorbidities of patients undergoing ASCT, transplant-related mortality reduced from 2.9% to 0.7% from 1998 to 2011. [41] One study of infection rates in ASCT found that 20.9% of all episodes of infection during ASCT were fever of unknown focus, with the majority of infections occurring during ASCT of high severity (93.3%). [42]

INFECTIONS IN MULTIPLE MYELOMA

Infections are an important cause of morbidity in patients with MM and a leading cause of death, with approximately 50% of early deaths in MM due to infection. [43] Therefore we believe it is important to present the most recent information regarding the statistics of patients. Overall, patients with MM have increased incidence of infection in the first few months of starting therapy with chemotherapeutic agents and in the last stage of the disease's progression. [44] As stated prior, clinical complications that increase the risk of infection are neutropenia, neurodegenerative disease, kidney failure, fractures, and other disease and treatment related comorbidities. [45]

We found 12 relevant articles discussing infectious complications of multiple myeloma patients using the search terms "multiple myeloma" and "infections" using the PubMed search database. We narrowed results to the English language only, full-text articles only, and articles published between January 1st 2008 to January 1st 2018. This covered 19,854 total number of

MM patients. The results of our search are detailed in Table 1. [46, 47, 48, 49, 50, 51, 52, 53, 54, 55, 56, 57]

Of the studies that reported age, the range of median ages was between 56 and 72, with 66.48 being the average age of all studies combined. It appeared that men were more frequently represented in the studies in all but one report. Bacterial infections were the most common types of infections reported in all studies. Pneumonia and bacteremia are the most common type of bacterial infections reported, and are typically caused by *Streptococcus pneumonia, Staphylococcus aureus,* and *Escherichia coli*; these results are similar to what has been reported in other cases and meta-analyses in the literature. [58] Other bacterial infections we noted included respiratory tract infection, blood stream infections, fever of unknown origin (FUO). Skin and soft tissue infections, osteomyelitis, pyelonephritis, cellulitis, meningitis, endocarditis, urinary tract infections. The types of viral infections seen in patients with MM included zoster, herpes simplex, herpes simplex dermatitis, herpes simplex ophthalmic, cytomegalovirus (CMV) infection, herpes viral infection NOS. The type of fungal infections seen in these patients included oral candidiasis, *Aspergillus*, esophageal candidiasis, *Candida* pneumonia, septicemia *Candida*, aspergillosis, *Pneumocystis carinii* pneumonia. Mortality rate was difficult to generalize given the different periods of time that each study was continued for with some reporting mortality during the period observed and some reporting mortality one year after the study was initially performed. However, rates ranged from 0.43% to 22.2%. The types of chemotherapeutic agents varied in each study with lenalidomide, thalidomide, and bortezomib being the most commonly reported agent. ASCT was also reported in a majority of the studies. Factors that were thought to be associated with increased risk of infections in patients with MM were neutropenia, increased serum creatinine indicating renal dysfunction, immunoparesis, anemia, hypercalcemia, elevated lactate dehydrogenase (LDH) level, and increased severity of disease based on the Durie-Salmon stage of disease.

Management of MM patients with prolonged and febrile neutropenia involves administration of prophylactic and empirical antibiotics; however, the choice of antibiotic therapy depends on the risk stratification of the individual patient. In low risk patients (duration of neutropenia is <1 week with no comorbid medical conditions), ciprofloxacin or levofloxacin are adequate, but in high risk patients (duration of neutropenia is >1 week with comorbid medical conditions) IV ceftazidime, IV piperacillin-tazobactam, or IV carbapenem can be given either alone or in combination with vancomycin or an aminoglycoside. Empirical antifungal therapy can be used in patients who have persistent fever despite using broad-spectrum antibiotics. Recombinant G-CSF as primary prophylaxis has been shown to improve quality of life and reduce the days of hospitalization, infectious complications, and incidence of chemotherapy interruptions. [60]

The overwhelming majority of studies show benefits for antibiotic prophylaxis in MM patients for infections, during chemotherapy, and during and after ASCT, but there are a few studies that do not. One study found antibacterial prophylaxis (ciprofloaxin) to be somewhat effective in MM patients undergoing chemotherapy and ASCT—while the rates of febrile neutropenia and bacteremia were higher in patients not receiving antibacterial prophylaxis, there was no difference in the frequency of other infections, hospital stay duration, and infection-related mortality between the group with and without prophylaxis. [61] Another study of 202 MM patients who underwent AHCT with or without ciprofloxacin prophylaxis found that febrile neutropenia, bacteremia, and pneumonia were significantly more common in patients without prophylaxis than those with. [62] Another study found that levofloxacin prophylaxis was associated with decreased risk of bloodstream infections and febrile neutropenia in patients with MM undergoing autologous HSCT. [63] Yet another study found that levofloxacin prophylaxis in MM patients being treated with bortezomib showed decreased severe infections compared to the control group. [64] Antibiotic prophylaxis was also shown to reduce incidence rates of febrile episodes, especially unexplained fever, in MM patients who underwent ASCT. [65] Another study looking at 356 MM patients undergoing AHCT found that antibacterial prophylaxis with ciprofloxacin significantly reduced the risk of febrile neutropenia, bacteremia, and pneumonia (although the frequency of other infections, infection-related mortality, and number of days from transplantation to discharge were not different between groups).

[66] Another study examining the role of antibacterial prophylaxis in preventing central line-associated blood stream infections in MM patients undergoing ASCT found that antibiotic prophylaxis reduced the risk of febrile neutropenia and risk of central line associated blood stream infections. [67] However, one study of 212 MM patients being treated with myelotoxic chemotherapy randomized to prophylactic ciprofloxacin, prophylactic trimethoprim-sulfamethoxazole (Bactrim), or observation found that infection incidence in the first 2 months were not significantly different ($p = 0.910$), that antibiotic prophylaxis did not decrease the incidence of serious infection (>grade 3 and/or hospitalization), and that antibiotic prophylaxis did not affect response to therapy or to overall survival. [68] Given this, the study advised that routine use of prophylactic antibiotics should be considered on a case-by-case basis after analyzing potential infection risks in MM individuals.

There are certain vaccines that are recommended as prophylaxis for individuals with MM given these individuals increased risk of infection. The Advisory Committee on Immunization Practices recommends that patients with MM should receive vaccination with PCV13 at diagnosis, followed by revaccination with PPV23 8 or more weeks later. [69] Patients 65 and older without other conditions should receive PCV13, followed by PPV23 within 6-12 months.

Other organizations are less clear with regards to recommendations on vaccination timing and schedule. The Naitonal Comprehensive Cancer Network recommends MM patients to "consider Pneumovax and influenza vaccine" without recommending a clear timing and schedule. [70] In short, many studies and organizations would recommend vaccination in MM patients for influenza, pneumococcal pneumonia, and H. influenza, though efficacy is not guaranteed. [71]

Conclusion

It is important to recognize the risks of infection and high incidence of infection-related mortality in MM patients, particularly with the advent of new and emerging therapies for this disease. We present a brief summary on the pathophysiology of MM, the current and emerging therapies for this disease, and the prevalence of infections in MM patients as well as strategies to manage and prevent these infections.

REFERENCES

[1] Gerecke C, Fuhrmann S, Strifler S, Schmidt-Hieber M, Einsele H, Knop S. The Diagnosis and Treatment of Multiple Myeloma. *Dtsch Arztebl Int*. 2016;113(27-28):470-6.

[2] Al-Farsi K. Multiple myeloma: an update. *Oman Med J*. 2013; 28(1):3-11.

[3] Pratt G, Goodyear O, Moss P. Immunodeficiency and immune-therapy in multiple myeloma. *Br J Haematol*. 2007; 138(5): 563–79.

[4] Blade J, Rosinol L. Renal, hematologic and infectious complications in multiple myeloma. *Best Pract Res Clin Haematol* 2005; 18(4); 635-52.

[5] Blimark C, Holmberg E, Mellqvist UH, et al. Multiple myeloma and infections: a population-based study on 9253 multiple myeloma patients. *Haematologica*. 2015;100(1):107-13.

[6] D'Agostino M, Boccadoro M, Smith EL. Novel Immunotherapies for Multiple Myeloma. *Curr Hematol Malig Rep*. 2017;12(4):344-357.

[7] Kazandjian D. Multiple myeloma epidemiology and survival: A unique malignancy. *Semin Oncol*. 2016;43(6):676-681.

[8] Brigle K, Rogers B. Pathobiology and Diagnosis of Multiple Myeloma. *Semin Oncol Nurs* 2017;33(3):225-236.

[9] Siegel RL, Miller KD, Jemal A. Cancer statistics, 2019. *CA Cancer J Clin* 2019;69(1):7-34.

[10] Kyle RA, Therneau TM, Rajkumar SV, Larson DR, Plevak MF, Melton LJ 3rd. Incidence of multiple myelma in Olmsted County, Minnesota: Trend over 6 decades. *Cancer* 2004; 101(11):2667-74.

[11] Cowan AJ, Allen C, Barac A, et al. Global Burden of Multiple Myeloma: A Systematic Analysis for the Global Burden of Disease Study 2016. *JAMA Oncol.* 2018;4(9):1221–1227.

[12] Banavali A, Neculiseanu E, Draksharam PL, et al. Findings of Multiple Myeloma in Afro-Caribbean Patients in the United States. *J Glob Oncol*. 2018;4(4):1-6.

[13] Kyle RA, Gertz MA, Witzig TE, et al. Review of 1027 patients with newly diagnosed multiple myeloma. *Mayo Clin Proc* 2003;78(1): 21-33.

[14] Blade J, Kyle RA. Multiple myeloma in young patients: clinical presentation and treatment approach. *Leuk Lymphoma* 1998;30(5-6):493-501.

[15] Rosenberg PS, Barker KA, Anderson WF. Future distribution of multiple myeloma in the United States by sex, age, and race/ ethnicity. *Blood*. 2015;125(2):410-2.

[16] American Cancer Society. Key Statistics About Multiple Myeloma. https://www.cancer.org/cancer/multiple-myeloma/about/key-statistics.html. Accessed February 18, 2019.

[17] Van Marion AMW, Lokhorst HM, van den Tweel JG. Pathology of multiple myeloma. *Current Diagnostic Pathology* 2003;9(5):322-7.

[18] Hameed A, Brady JJ, Dowling P, Clynes M, O'Gorman P. Bone disease in multiple myeloma: pathophysiology and management. *Cancer Growth Metastasis*. 2014;7:33-42.

[19] Kasper DL, Fauci AS, Hauser SL, Longo DL, Jameson J, Loscalzo J. (2015). Harrison's principles of internal medicine (19th edition.). New York: McGraw Hill Education. Kasper, Dennis L et al. Harrison's Principles of Internal Medicine

[20] Fairfield H, Falank C, Avery L, Reagan MR. Multiple myeloma in the marrow: pathogenesis and treatments. *Ann N Y Acad Sci*. 2016;1364(1):32-51.

[21] Seidl S, Kaufmann H, Drach J. New insights into the pathophysiology of multiple myeloma. *Lancet Oncol* 2003;4(9):557-63.

[22] Silbermann R, Roodman GD. Myeloma bone disease: Pathophysiology and management. *Journal of Bone Oncology* 2013; 2(2):59-9.

[23] Pratt G, Goodyear O, Moss P. Immunodeficiency and immune-therapy in multiple myeloma. *British Journal of Haematology* 2007.

[24] Rutella S, Locatelli F. Targeting multiple-myeloma-induced immune dysfunction to improve immunotherapy outcomes. *Clin Dev Immunol.* 2012;2012:196063.

[25] M. Rossi, C. Botta, P. Correale, P. Tassone, and P. Tagliaferri, "Immunologic microenvironment and personalized treatment in multiple myeloma," *Expert Opinion on Biological Therapy,* vol. 13, no. 1, supplement, pp. S83–S93, 2013.

[26] Yang WC, Lin SF. Mechanisms of Drug Resistance in Relapse and Refractory Multiple Myeloma. *Biomed Res Int.* 2015;2015:341430.

[27] Pellom ST, Dudimah DF, Thounaojam MC, Sayers TJ, Shanker A. Modulatory effects of bortezomib on host immune cell functions. *Immunotherapy*. 2015;7(9):1011-22.

[28] Nucci M, Anaissie E. Infections in Patients with Multiple Myleloma in the Era of High-Dose Therapy and Novel Agents. *Clin Infectious Diseases* 2009;49(8):1211-25.

[29] Mateos MV, Hernández JM, Hernández MT, Gutiérrez NC, Palomera L, Fuertes M, Díaz-Mediavilla J, Lahuerta JJ, Terol MJ, Sureda A, Bargay J, Ribas P, Arriba F, de, Alegre A, Oriol A, Carrera D, García-Laraña J, García-Sanz R, Bladé J, Prósper F, Mateo G, Esseltine DL, San Miguel JF. Bortezomib plus melphalan and prednisone in elderly untreated patients with multiple myeloma: results of a multicenter phase 1/2 study. *Blood.* 2006;108:2165–2172.

[30] Valković T, Gačić V, Ivandić J, et al. Infections in Hospitalised Patients with Multiple Myeloma: Main Characteristics and Risk Factors. *Turk J Haematol.* 2015;32(3):234-42.

[31] Zhu YX, Kortuem KM, Stewart AK. Molecular mechanism of action of immune-modulatory drugs thalidomide, lenalidomide and pomalidomide in multiple myeloma. *Leuk Lymphoma.* 2012; 54(4):683-7.

[32] Chen M, Zhao Y, Xu C et al. Immunomodulatory drugs and the risk of serious infection in multiple myeloma: systematic review and meta-

analysis of randomized and observational studies. *Annals of Hematology* 2018;97(6):925-44.

[33] Offidani M, Savini A, Corvatta L, et al. Infection Complications in Patients with Multiple Myeloma Treated with New-Drug Combinations Including Thalidomide. *Blood* 2009;114:2828.

[34] Richardson P, Mitsiades C, Schlossman R, et al. The treatment of relapsed and refractory multiple myeloma. *Hematology Am Soc Hematol Educ Program* 2007;317-23.

[35] Facon T, Mary JY, Hulin C, et al. Melphalan and prednisone plus thalidomide versus melphalan and prednisone alone or reduced-intensity autologous stem cell transplantation in elderly patients with multiple myeloma (IFM 99-06): a randomized trial. *Lancet* 2007;370(9594):1209-18.

[36] Koniarczyk HL, Ferraro C, Miceli T. Hematopoietic Stem Cell Transplantation for Multiple Myeloma. *Seminars in Oncology Nursing* 2017;33(3):265-78.

[37] Gertz MA, Dingli D. How we manage autologous stem cell transplantation for patients with multiple myeloma. *Blood.* 2014;124(6):882-90.

[38] Harousseau JL, Moreau P. Autologous Hematopoietic Stem-Cell Transplantation for Multiple Myeloma. *N Engl J Med* 2009; 360: 2645-54.

[39] Rajkumar SV, Kumar S. Multiple Myeloma: Diagnosis and Treatment. *Mayo Clin Proc*. 2016;91(1):101-19.

[40] Mahajan S, Tandon N, Kumar S. The evolution of stem-cell transplantation in multiple myeloma. *Ther Adv Hematol*. 2018;9 (5):123-133.

[41] Savani BN, Mukherjee A, Savani GT, et al. Utilization trend and in-hospital complications of autologous hematopoietic stem cell transplantation in multiple myeloma in the United States: 13 years perspective. *Blood* 2014; 124: 3978.

[42] Teh BW, Harrison SJ, Worth LJ, et al. Risks, severity and timing of infections in patients with multiple myeloma: a longitudinal cohort

study in the era of immunomodulatory drug therapy. *British Journal of Haematology* 2015;171(1):100-8.

[43] Teh, BW, Harrison, SJ, Pellegrini, M, Thursky, KA, Worth, LJ, Slavin, MA. Changing treatment paradigms for patients with plasma cell myeloma: impact upon immune determinants of infection. *Blood Rev* 2014; 28: 75– 86.

[44] Ying L, YinHui T, Yunliang Z, Sun H. Lenalidomide and the risk of serious infection in patients with multiple myeloma: a systematic review and meta-analysis. *Oncotarget.* 2017;8(28):46593-46600.

[45] Ying L, YinHui T, Yunliang Z, Sun H. Lenalidomide and the risk of serious infection in patients with multiple myeloma: a systematic review and meta-analysis. *Oncotarget.* 2017;8(28):46593-46600.

[46] Blimark C, Holmberg E, Mellqvist UH, et al. Multiple myeloma and infections: a population-based study on 9253 multiple myeloma patients. *Haematologica.* 2015;100(1):107-13.

[47] Offidani M, Corvatta L, Polloni C, et al. Infectious complications in patients with multiple myeloma treated with new drug combinations containing thalidomide. *Leuk Lymphoma.* 2011;52(5):776-85.

[48] Chanan-Khan A, Sonneveld P, Schuster MW, et al. Analysis of herpes zoster events among bortezomib-treated patients in the phase III APEX study. *J Clin Oncol.* 2008;26(29):4784-90.

[49] Caravita T, Offidani M, Siniscalchi A, et al. Infection complications in an unselected cohort of patients with multiple myeloma treated with lenalidomide complications. *Eur J Haematol.* 2012;89(3):276-7.

[50] Kristinsson SY, Tang M, Pfeiffer RM, et al. Monoclonal gammopathy of undetermined significance and risk of infections: a population-based study. *Haematologica.* 2012;97(6):854-8.

[51] Ying L, YinHui T, Yunliang Z, Sun H. Lenalidomide and the risk of serious infection in patients with multiple myeloma: a systematic review and meta-analysis. *Oncotarget.* 2017;8(28):46593-46600.

[52] Huang CT, Liu CJ, Ko PS, et al. Risk factors and characteristics of blood stream infections in patients with newly diagnosed multiple myeloma. *BMC Infect Dis.* 2017;17(1):33. Published 2017 Jan 6.

[53] Park H, Youk J, Kim HR. Infectious complications in multiple myeloma receiving autologous stem cell transplantation in the past 10 years. *Internationl Journal of Hematology*. 2017;106(6):801-10.

[54] Valković T, Gačić V, Ivandić J, et al. Infections in Hospitalised Patients with Multiple Myeloma: Main Characteristics and Risk Factors. *Turk J Haematol*. 2015;32(3):234-42.

[55] Teh BW, Harrison SJ, Slavin MA, Worth LJ. Epidemiology of bloodstream infections in patients with myeloma receiving current era therapy. *Eur J Haematol*. 2017;98(2):149-53.

[56] Sørrig R, Klausen TW, Salomo M, et al. Risk factors for bloodstream infections in multiple myeloma: A population-based study of 1154 patients in Denmark. *Eur J Haematol*. 2018; 101(1):21-7.

[57] Teh BW, Harrison SJ, Worth LJ, et al. Risks, severity, and timing of infections in patients with multiple myeloma: a longitudinal cohort study in the era of immunomodulatory drug therapy. *Br J Haematol*. 2015;171(1):100-8.

[58] Nucci M, Anaissie E. Infections in Patients with Multiple Myeloma in the Era of High-Dose Therapy and Novel Agents. *Clin Infect Diseases*. 2009;49(8):1211-25.

[59] Al-Jasser AM, Al-Anazi KA. Infections in Patients with Multiple Myeloma in the Era of Novel Agents and Stem Cell Therapies. *Intech Open*. 2018.

[60] Al-Jasser AM, Al-Anazi KA. Infections in Patients with Multiple Myeloma in the Era of Novel Agents and Stem Cell Therapies. *Intech Open*. 2018.

[61] Shargian-Alon L, Vaxman J, Rozvoski U, et al. Antibacterial Prophylaxis Reduces the Risk of Bacteremia in Patients with Multiple Myeloma and Lymphoma Undergoing High-Dose Chemotherapy and Autologous Stem Cell Transplantation. *Clinical Lymphome, Myeloma & Leukemia*. 2016;16. S77-8.

[62] Yeshurun M, Vaxman I, Shargian L, et al. Antibacterial prophylaxis with ciprofloxacin for patients with multiple myeloma and lymphoma undergoing autologous haematopoietic cell transplantation: a quasi-

experimental single-centre before-after study. *Clinical Microbiology and Infection.* 2018;24(7):749-54.

[63] Satlin MJ, Vardhana S, Soave R, et al. Impact of Prophylactic Levofloxacin on Rates of Bloodstream Infection and Fever in Neutropenic Patients with Multiple Myeloma Undergoing Autologous Hematopoietic Stem Cell Transplantation. *Biol Blood Marrow Transplant*. 2015;21(10):1808-14.

[64] Jung SH, Kang, SJ, Jang, HC. Effect of levofloxacin prophylaxis for prevention of severe infections in multiple myeloma patients receiving bortezomib-containing regiments. *Int J Hematol.* 2014; 100(5):473-7.

[65] Sohn BS, Yoon DH, Kim S, et al. The role of prophylactic antimicrobials during autologous stem cell transplantation: a single-center experience. *Eur J Clin Microbiol Infect Dis.* 2012;31(7):1653-61.

[66] Vaxman J, Rozovsky U, Shargian L, et al. Antibacterial Prophylaxis Reduces the Risk of Bacteremia and Febrile Neutropenia in Patients with Multiple Myeloma and Lymphoma Undergoing High-Dose Chemotherapy and Autologous Hematopoietic Cell Transplantation. *Biology of Blood and Marrow Transplantation.* 2017;23(3):S201.

[67] Watts N, Chodavarapu A, Rahman M, et al. The Role of Antibacterial Prophylaxis in Preventing Central Line-Associated Bloodstream Infections (CLABSIs) in Multiple Myeloma Patients Undergoing an Autologous Stem Cell Transplant. *Biology of Blood and Marrow Transplantation.* 2017;23(3):S199-200.

[68] Vesole DH, Oken MM, Heckler C, et al. Oral Antibiotic Prophylaxis of Early Infection in Multiple Myeloma: A URCC/ECOG Phase III Study. *Blood.* 2010; 116:3017.

[69] Bonten MJ, Huijts SM, Bolkenbaas M, et al. Polysaccharide conjugate vaccine against pneumococcal pneumonia in adults. *N Engl J Med.* 2015;372:1114-25.

[70] Anderson KC, Alsina M, Atanackovic D, et al. Multiple Myeloma version 2. 2016: clinical practice guideliens in oncology. *J Natl Compr Canc Netw.* 2015;13:1398-1435.

[71] Al-Farsi K. Multiple myeloma: an update. *Oman Med* J. 2013;28:3-11.

In: Horizons in Cancer Research. Volume 73 ISBN: 978-1-53616-273-8
Editor: Hiroto S. Watanabe

Chapter 6

PLANT-DERIVED LECTINS: A REVIEW OF THEIR STATUS AS ALTERNATIVES TO ANTICANCER CHEMOTHERAPY

Leydianne L. S. Patriota[1], Jéssica S. Brito[1], Dalila B. M. Ramos[1], Thamara F. Procópio[1], Patrícia M. G. Paiva[1], Emmanuel V. Pontual[2], Cristiane M. L. Melo[3] and Thiago H. Napoleão[1,*]

[1]Departamento de Bioquímica,
Universidade Federal de Pernambuco, Recife, Pernambuco, Brazil
[2]Departamento de Morfologia e Fisiologia Animal,
Universidade Federal Rural de Pernambuco,
Recife, Pernambuco, Brazil
[3]Departamento de Antibióticos, Universidade Federal de Pernambuco,
Recife, Pernambuco, Brazil

[*] Corresponding Author's Email: thiagohn86@yahoo.com.br.

ABSTRACT

Plants are rich sources of compounds with varied structures and potent biological effects against diseases, including cancer. Many studies have been performed to investigate plant-derived compounds with the ability to impair tumor formation or control cancer progression such as lectins (carbohydrate-binding proteins). This review discusses the *in vitro* and/or *in vivo* effects of these bioactive proteins from plants against cancer cells or models. Lectins interfere with cell growth and survival by binding to specific membrane receptors or internalization via endocytosis. In both cases, they can block the pathways involved in cell growth and survival (e.g., PI3K/Akt/mTOR, ERK, and NF-κB signaling), induce oxidative stress, trigger apoptosis through the induction of an imbalance of pro-apoptotic and anti-apoptotic proteins and/or the activation of death receptors, induce autophagy-related gene expression, and cause necrosis. Although some lectins have been studied in clinical trials, there are many others that deserve attention. The current study indicates such proteins that have a promising future as new anticancer drugs.

Keywords: natural compounds, antineoplastic activity, plant proteins, action mechanisms

INTRODUCTION

Cancer is the name given to a set of more than 100 diseases that have in common the disordered growth of cells. As one of the leading causes of morbidity and mortality, it is a major global public health problem. Cancer can arise in any organ and result in distinct clinical manifestations; the characteristics of neoplastic cells include self-sufficiency for growth signals, insensitivity to anti-growth signals, stimulation of local angiogenesis, and, frequently, an ability to escape apoptosis (Aunan et al., 2017).

From the 2012 GLOBOCAN project, 14.1 million cases of cancer were estimated globally; 7.4 million cases in men and 6.7 million in women. This number is expected to increase to 24 million by 2035 (Ferlay et al., 2015). According to the World Health Organization (2018), approximately 8.8

million deaths were attributable to cancer in 2015, corresponding to one death in every six patients.

Cancer originates from a series of successive mutations that lead to the loss of pro-apoptotic protein functions or an increase in the expression of antiapoptotic genes, causing the cells to develop mechanisms to evade apoptosis and favor continuous tumor growth. The cancer may be benign – when cells remain localized and damage only the organ in which they are located – or malignant. In malignant tumors, the cells lose differentiation and adhesion capabilities, and develop the ability to invade and colonize diverse tissues and organs, a phenomenon known as metastasis (Faheina-Martins et al., 2012).

The mechanisms of apoptosis evasion in neoplastic cells arise from the increased expression of antiapoptotic genes or the loss of function of pro-apoptotic proteins, which are codified by proto-oncogenes that become oncogenes owing to genetic mutations (translocation, amplification, or punctual mutation). In addition, uncontrolled cell division and tumor growth may be triggered by a lack of tumor suppressor genes, such as *p53*, which regulate cell cycle arrest and apoptosis in response to DNA damage (Aunan et al., 2017; Yue et al., 2017).

Despite major advances in our understanding of cancer biology, further efforts are needed to identify new therapies capable of overcoming resistance, recurrence, and metastasis. The major challenge is the genetic diversity of cancer; the interactions between heterogeneous tumor cells, stroma, and immune cells are also of importance (Derbal, 2017). In addition, the chemotherapeutics currently used may lead to various and severe side effects and the number of reports of cancers resistant to traditional therapies is increasing (Powathil et al., 2014; Pan et al., 2016). The discovery of new medicinal agents from plants, including bioactive proteins such as lectins and protease inhibitors (Yau et al., 2015; Srikanth and Chen, 2016), may minimize the impact of drug resistance and toxicity (Al-Mamun et al., 2016; Arul and Subramanian, 2013).

In this review, we have first provided an initial overview on cancer and the currently available anticancer agents; subsequently, we have focused on the roles of lectins from plants as alternative anticancer agents. We have also discussed the mechanisms of action involved in the anticancer activity of these proteins.

TYPES OF CELL DEATH

The dysregulation of the control of cell death, in positive or negative direction, is the basis of several pathologies, including cancer, autoimmunity, and neurodegeneration. Different types of cell death have distinct morphological characteristics and physiological processes; however, these factors exhibit complex interactions.

Apoptosis is the most well-characterized form of programmed cell death and has been extensively investigated. It involves the controlled disassembly of intracellular components, which prevents inflammation and damage to surrounding cells, and is characterized by chromatin condensation, nuclear fragmentation, shrinkage, pseudopodia retraction, the formation of apoptotic bodies, and phagocytosis by neighboring cells (Kumar et al., 2007; McIlwain et al., 2013). Caspases, a group of cysteine proteases, are the main promoters of apoptotic cell death. The various apoptotic pathways can be distinguished by the initiator caspase and adaptors involved (McIlwain et al., 2013; Parrish et al., 2013).

The intrinsic (mitochondrial) pathway, the predominant mechanism of apoptosis, results in increased mitochondrial permeability and the release of pro-apoptotic molecules within the cytoplasm, which is controlled by the balance between the pro- and antiapoptotic members of the Bcl family of proteins. Growth factors and other signs of survival stimulate the production of antiapoptotic proteins, mainly Bcl-2 and Bcl-x, which control mitochondrial permeability and prevent the extravasation of mitochondrial proteins. When cells are deprived of survival signals or their DNA is damaged, lesion or stress sensors are activated. These sensors are also members of the Bcl family and include the proteins Bim, Bid, and Bad, which subsequently activate two critical pro-apoptotic effectors, Bax and Bak; these proteins insert into the mitochondrial membrane and create channels to allow proteins from the inner mitochondrial membrane to extravase to the cytoplasm. The sensors can also bind to Bcl-2 and Bcl-x and block their functions. When released into the cytosol, cytochrome c binds to the Apaf-1 (apoptosis-activating factor-1) protein to form the apoptosome. This complex can bind to caspase-9 and trigger the caspase activation cascade (Kumar et al., 2007).

The extrinsic apoptosis pathway is initiated by the involvement of plasma membrane death receptors, which are members of the TNF receptor family and contain a cytoplasmic domain known as the "death domain." Examples include TNF receptor type 1 (TNFR1) and the related protein Fas, which binds to the Fas-ligand (FasL) and forms a binding site for an adapter protein called Fas-associated death domain (FADD), which in turn binds to pro-caspase-10 and initiates the caspase activation cascade. Once a triggering caspase is cleaved to its active form, executioner caspases, such as caspase-3 and -6, affect many cellular components, degrading the structural components of the nuclear matrix and promoting the fragmentation of the nucleus (Kumar et al., 2007).

Autophagy is a lysosomal-dependent process that degrades molecules from whole organelles. It is a cellular mechanism for the clearance of components of excessively damaged eukaryotic cells, which can lead to both pro-survival and pro-death effects (Shi et al., 2013). During autophagy, an insulation membrane forms in the cytoplasm, engulfing the cytosolic charge to create an autophagosome. Mature autophagosomes fuse with lysosomes, which leads to the digestion of the engulfed material and allows the macromolecules to be recycled. Autophagy is a complex process performed by autophagy-related genes (ATG) and their respective proteins (for example ATG4, ATG5, and ATG6). Autophagy is crucial to many processes, including development, immunity, and cellular aging (Choi et al., 2013; Shibutani et al., 2015).

Necrosis and necroptosis are forms of cell death that are characterized by the distension of the organelles and the consequent loss of cell membrane integrity and release of intracellular constituents in the extracellular space, which may lead to inflammation. After acute cell injury, necrosis apparently occurs in a disorderly fashion. However, recent studies have shown that necrosis can also be induced by specific stimuli and programmed by a signaling pathway, this type of death called necroptosis (Wallach et al., 2014). The characteristic features of necrotic cells include a more translucent cytoplasm, swelling of cytoplasmic organelles, the condensation of chromatin in circumscribed and irregular patches, and an increase in cell volume that culminates in mechanical rupture of the plasma membrane. Necrotic cells do not fragment into discrete bodies, nor do their nuclei, which accumulate in necrotic tissues (Kepp et al., 2011). Necrosis is considered as a passive event resulting from a cellular extrinsic stimulus, such as infection by pathogens (Blériot and Lecuit, 2016).

Other forms of non-apoptotic death are pyrocytosis, caspase-independent cell death, and mitotic catastrophe. These may contribute to physiological cell death in cases of both proficient and deficient apoptosis. Understanding the mechanism of caspase-independent cell death may allow the development of manipulations with varied therapeutic uses, such as cancer and autoimmune diseases (Tait et al., 2014).

ACTION MECHANISMS OF ANTICANCER AGENTS

The final goal of chemotherapy agents is the induction of cell death in tumor cells. This is a complex process in which many different genes are involved, especially tumor suppressor genes and oncogenes (Aunan et al., 2017). p53 is a tumor suppressor protein that regulates cell cycle arrest and apoptosis in response to DNA damage (Yue et al., 2017). DNA damage indirectly results in p53 activation via kinases and leads to cell cycle arrest. Mutations within the *p53* gene have been observed in human cancers (Reinhardt and Schumacher, 2012; Yue et al., 2017). DNA-damaging drugs tested in clinical trials induce cell death through interference with p53; for example, disulfiram depletes mutant p53 and chetomin, leading to restoration of wild-type p53 transcriptional activity (Parrales and Iwakuma, 2015).

As previously discussed, the caspases are regulated by the Bcl family of proteins. ABT-737 and its clinical analog ABT-263 (navitoclax) are small molecules that prevent the binding of pro-apoptotic Bcl family members (Hata et al., 2015).

The phosphatidylinositol-3-kinase (PI3K)/protein kinase B (Akt/PKB) and the mammalian target of rapamycin (mTOR) signaling pathways are interconnected to such an extent that they can be regarded as a single pathway, the PI3K/Akt/mTOR pathway, which is crucial to many aspects of cell growth (LoPiccolo et al., 2008). The activation of this pathway results in competitive growth advantages, metastatic competence, and stimulation of angiogenesis. Thus, this pathway has been considered as one of the most attractive targets for the development of specific PI3K, Akt, and mTOR inhibitors as anticancer agents (Porta et al., 2014). The examples include the Akt inhibitors, perifosine and PX-866, and the mTOR inhibitors rapamycin, CCI-779, and RAD-001 (LoPiccolo et al., 2008).

The RAS-RAF-MEK-ERK pathway (ERK signaling) is an evolutionary conserved signaling cascade that transmits signals from the cell surface receptors to promote proliferation and survival (Matallanas et al., 2011). As components of the ERK signaling cascade are frequently mutated in cancer, this prompted the development of small-molecule inhibitors targeted to the components of ERK signaling for use as cancer therapeutics, such as the RAF inhibitors vemurafenib (Zelboraf; Genentech/Plexxikon) and dabrafenib (Tafinlar; GlaxoSmithKline) and the MEK inhibitor trametinib (GSK) (Samatar and Poulikakos, 2014).

Nuclear factor kappa-light-chain-enhancer of activated B cells (NF-κB) is a signaling molecule; a significant number of human cancers have constitutive NF-κB activity, which promotes tumor cell proliferation, suppresses apoptosis, and stimulates angiogenesis (Wade et al., 2013). Bortezomib is a NF-κB inhibitor that has been approved by the Federal Drug Administration (FDA) and the European regulatory agency (EMEA) for the treatment of multiple myeloma (Wade et al., 2013).

Modulation of the cell cycle also contributes to chemotherapy resistance. The cyclin-dependent kinases (CDKs), together with regulatory proteins called cyclins, drive the cell through the cycle; thus, they are rational therapeutic targets. CDK inhibitors, such as flavopiridol and olomoucine, block specific interactions of cyclin complexes, which can induce apoptosis (Dickson and Schwartz, 2009; Otto and Sicinski, 2017).

Furthermore, reactive oxygen species (ROS) kill cells by causing oxidative damage to lipids, proteins, and DNA. Doxorubicin (DOX) exerts antitumor action on DNA through modification of the mechanism of repair mediated by topoisomerase II, as well as through the release of free radicals. This occurs when DOX is oxidized into an unstable metabolite which, upon return to the reduced state, releases ROS. One of the major drawbacks related to the use of DOX is cardiotoxicity (Faraji et al., 2016).

Initially developed as an analog of folic acid, methotrexate (MTX) was one of the first chemotherapy agents used clinically. It functions through the inhibition of DNA replication and repair, which slows cell proliferation and leads to cell death. It is used for the treatment of acute leukemias and lymphomas (Thomas et al., 2015). One of the main side effects of MTX, which restricts its clinical use, is hepatotoxicity (Mehrzadi et al., 2018).

Over the past 20 years, patients diagnosed with solid and hematological cancers have had access to a greater number of therapeutic options. Many of them have experienced better overall survival and long-term remission since the introduction of new classes of cancer agents. However, these new agents and their combinations have come with additional toxicities and, as the liver is responsible for the metabolism of the majority of these drugs, hepatotoxicity usually occurs during treatments (Dhanasekaran and Kwo, 2017).

Lectins

Lectins are proteins that interact with carbohydrates in a specific and reversible way, and are found abundantly in nature and isolated from bacteria, fungi, animals, and plants. These proteins have at least one non-catalytic domain that is capable of reversible binding to simple carbohydrates (monosaccharides and disaccharides), complex oligosaccharides (including the glycoconjugate portion of glycoconjugates) and/or polysaccharides (Hamid et al., 2013). The presence of at least two carbohydrate binding sites in the structure of a lectin confers agglutination properties. The hemagglutination assay (Figure 1), in which the capacity of interaction between the lectin and carbohydrates of the erythrocyte surface is evaluated, is the most commonly used method for lectin detection (Santos et al., 2013).

The ability of lectins to bind to carbohydrates on the cell surface can trigger intracellular responses, resulting in a range of biological properties that have been exploited for biotechnological and medicinal purposes. Among the biological activities described for lectins, insecticidal (Lima et al., 2017), antiviral (Sato et al., 2012), antifungal (Silva et al., 2018), antibacterial (Moura et al., 2015), antiangiogenic (Ambasta et al., 2015), antinociceptive (Campos et al., 2016), anti-inflammatory (Campos et al., 2016), mitogenic (Singh et al., 2015), and immunomodulatory (Patriota et al., 2017) effects have been highlighted, as well as antineoplastic and antitumor activities, which are discussed further below. In addition, lectins have been studied as tools to assist the diagnosis and prognosis of diseases and have been used in histochemical probes owing to their ability for differential tissue and cell recognition (Santos et al., 2014; Silva et al., 2016).

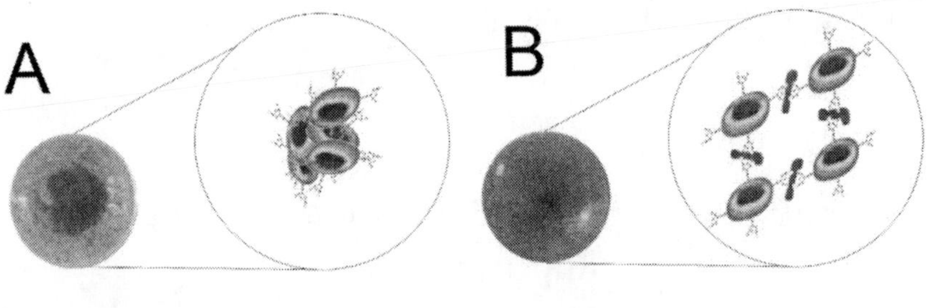

Figure 1. Schematic representation of the hemagglutinating activity of lectins. (A) In the absence of lectins, the erythrocytes precipitate in the well of a V-bottomed microplate. (B). In the presence of lectins, a network forms between the lectin (in gray) and the carbohydrates of the erythrocyte surface and there is no precipitation. The agglutination can be observed visually by naked eye.

As lectins can inhibit proliferation and induce the death of tumor cells, they are naturally good candidates for anticancer agents. In human case studies, it has been demonstrated that they can function as an alternative cancer therapy (Liu et al., 2010; Yau et al., 2015; Estrada-Martínez et al., 2017). Lectins may exert toxicity to cancer cells through different mechanisms, such as the induction of apoptosis, autophagy, necrosis, or the inhibition of cell growth.

Glycosylation of the cell surface proteins play a key role in cell development, signaling, interaction, proliferation, differentiation, and migration. Cancer cells are phenotypically different from normal cells with respect to the pattern of carbohydrates expressed on the cell surface. These changes may result from the altered activity of glycosyltransferases and glycosidases and are seen in glycolipids and glycoproteins (Ghazarian et al., 2011; Christiansen et al., 2014). The change in glycosylation is a universal feature of tumor cells, with certain glycans being well-known markers of tumor progression. One of the first pieces of evidence that altered glycosylation was a characteristic of cancer was the discovery that some lectins from plants improve the specific agglutination capacity of these cells (Varki et al., 2017). These differences in the patterns of glycosylation allow the lectins to distinguish between normal and cancer cells (Tozawa-Ono et al., 2017).

Anticancer Lectins from Plants and Their Mechanism of Action

Lectins have been isolated from a large variety of plant tissues and organs, such as flowers, leave, seeds, stems, bulbs, fruits, bark, wood, and root (Paiva et al., 2011; Dias et al., 2015). Plant lectins induce toxicity to cancer cells via different mechanisms (Figure 2), which are usually initiated through interactions with specific receptors, both glycosylated and unglycosylated, in the membrane of cancer cells; subsequently, the lectins can activate the signaling cascades linked to cell death and/or be internalized via endocytosis, reaching different compartments and activate other death cascades (Gabor et al., 2001; Yau et al., 2015). Lectins promote cell death through the modulation of important mechanisms involved in cell growth and survival (blocking PI3K/Akt/mTOR, NF-κB, ERK signaling pathways), oxidative stress (stimulation of ROS release), cell cycle (upregulation of p53 and induction of cell cycle arrest), intrinsic apoptosis (upregulation of pro-apoptotic proteins and downregulation of antiapoptotic proteins, activation of caspases, and promotion of the release of cytochrome c); extrinsic apoptosis (release of death receptors such as Fas and TNF); autophagy (upregulation of ATG and their respective proteins), and mitochondrial function (decrease in membrane potential and loss of membrane integrity). Several lectins exert different forms of antitumor action against various cell types.

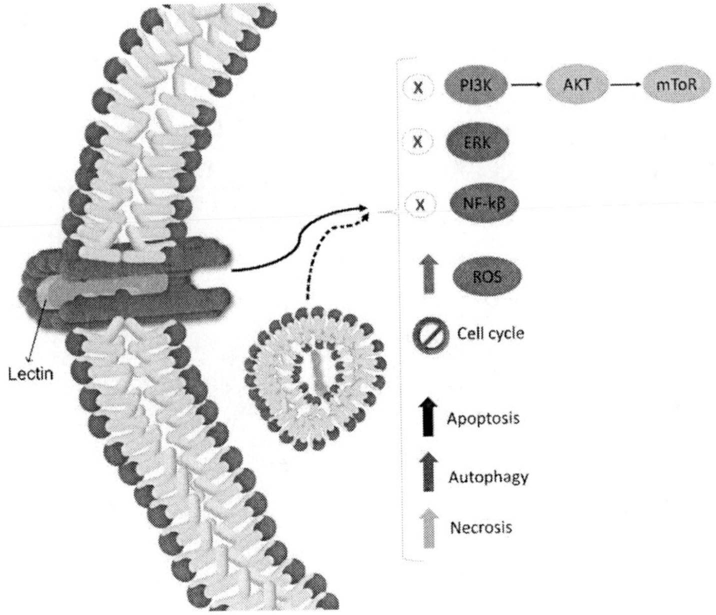

Figure 2. Mechanisms involved in the toxicity of plant lectins to cancer cells. Lectinas can interact with specific receptors at cell membrane and activate the signaling cascades linked to cell death (solid arrow). Alternatively, lectins can be internalized via endocytosis reaching different compartments and activate the death cascades (dashed arrows).

AAG is a lectin isolated from the seeds of *Abrus precatorius* that shows specificity towards galactose or galactose-containing carbohydrates. It is a tetrameric glycoprotein of 134 kDa composed of two nonidentical polypeptide chains (A and B) and belongs to type II RIPs family (Tahirov et al., 1995). Abrin is a hetero-dimeric glycoprotein with a mass of 63 kDa, which belongs to the RIPs II family and shares a high degree of sequence similarity with AAG (Bagaria et al., 2006). Abrin and AAG are composed of a toxic subunit, the A chain, and a galactose-binding B chain; a single disulfide bond covalently links the two chains. Abrin is extremely toxic to eukaryotic cells, whereas AAG has low toxicity (Liu et al., 2000). Despite this, abrin is much more toxic to some transformed cell lines than to normal cells and is therefore attractive as a potential anticancer agent (Mejía and Prisecaru, 2005). The antitumor activity of abrin has been reported in *in vitro* (Bhutia et al., 2016) and *in vivo* (Ramnath et al., 2009) conditions.

Abrin binds to cell-surface receptors containing terminal galactose through the B subunit and induces apoptosis in human leukemic T-cell lymphoblast cells (Jurkat) through the intrinsic mitochondrial pathway and caspase-3 activation, inducing mitochondrial membrane potential damage and ROS production (Narayanan et al., 2004). Abrin-derived peptides, obtained through tryptic digestion, induced apoptosis by targeting mitochondria in human cervical cancer (HeLa) cells. Unlike the parent lectin, the activity of the peptides was independent of sugar binding; after penetration of the cell membrane and induction of apoptosis, they target mitochondria. Thus, the authors highlighted that this peptide fraction was a source of mitochondria-penetrating peptides with possible therapeutic activity against in cancer cells (Bhutia et al., 2009b). Abrin-derived peptides were also found to reduce the expression of Bcl-2, increase the expression of Bax, and activate caspase-3 through the release of cytochrome c in Dalton's lymphoma cells (DL), resulting in the functional alteration of the mitochondria and induction of apoptotic responses (Bhutia et al., 2009a). Previously heat-denatured abrin at non-toxic doses significantly decreased the number of lymphoma cells in DL tumor-bearing mice (Ghosh and Maiti, 2007). The combination of ABRaA-VEGF121 (a fusion recombinant protein composed of VEGF isoform 121 and abrin A chain) and an immunostimulatory cytokine (IL-12) inhibited the growth of murine melanoma (B16-F10) cells and led to total tumor cure in approximately 20% of mice (Ciomber et al., 2013).

The anticancer effects of AAG have been evaluated in several tumor models, where this lectin inhibited the growth of tumors in experimental animals, such as human hepatocellular carcinoma (HepG2). AAG induced apoptosis in HepG2 cells in a dose- and time-dependent manner. AGG-treated HepG2 cells exhibited an increase in the activity of caspase 3, 7, 8, and 9 and a sharp decrease in the Bcl-2/Bax ratio (Mukhopadhyay et al., 2014).

More recently, it was shown that AAG induced both intrinsic and extrinsic apoptosis through ROS activation in human breast cancer cells (MCF-7, MDA-MB-231, MDA-MB-157, and T47D), but induced minimal toxicity to normal breast cells. Moreover, the inhibition of Akt by AAG plays a central regulatory role in the ability of this lectin to induce apoptosis and inhibit angiogenesis in these cell lines (Bhutia et al., 2016).

Concanavalin A (ConA) is a lectin from the seeds of *Canavalia ensifomis* (jack bean) with specificity for mannose/glucose, and is a homotetramer with a mass of 112 kDa (each subunit of 26.5 kDa), belonging to the legume lectins family (Sumner and Howell, 1936). ConA is widely reported to have apoptosis and autophagy-inducing properties, which makes it a potential antineoplastic agent for cancer therapeutics (Li et al., 2011a). Studies reported that ConA induced apoptosis in human melanoma (A375) cells and murine macrophage PU5-1.8 cells. This lectin can also lead to the potential collapse of mitochondrial membrane potential, cytochrome c release, and caspase activation, which eventually triggers mitochondria-mediated apoptosis in both A375 and HepG2 cells (Suen et al., 2000; Li et al., 2011a; Liu et al., 2009d). ConA was also able to inhibit the growth of MCF-7 cells in a dose- and time-dependent manner (IC_{50} = 15 μg/mL), induced apoptosis through an increase in the activities of caspase-3 and caspase-9, the release of cytochrome c from mitochondria, the upregulation of Bax and Bid, the downregulation of Bcl-2 and Bcl-XL, and the upregulation of p53. ConA also reduced ERK signaling and an antitumor effect was demonstrated *in vivo* (Shi et al., 2014).

In glioblastoma cells (U87), ConA up-regulated expression of COX-2 and down-regulates Akt expression. In addition, ConA induced autophagy by the upregulation of ATG3 and ATG12 (Pratt et al., 2012; Pratt and Annabi, 2014). The inhibition of Akt expression was also involved in the induction of apoptosis by ConA in ovarian cancer cells (SKOV3) by rendering the ratio of Bax/Bcl-2 (Amin et al., 2007).

ConA treatment reduced the expression of PI3K/AKT/mTOR pathway members and induced the ERK pathway in HeLa cells, activating autophagy (Pratt and Annabi, 2014). ConA was also able to induce autophagy in BALB/c hepatoma cells (ML-1) via a mitochondrially-mediated pathway: it binds to the mannose residues present in cell membrane glycoproteins and is internalized to the mitochondria via clathrin-mediated endocytosis, initiating autophagy (Chang et al., 2007).

The antiproliferative activity of ConA was also studied in human leukemia cell lines (MOLT-4 and HL-60). It was revealed that ConA was markedly cytotoxic to these cell lines, which exhibited the morphological characteristic of apoptosis, showing a low concentration of apoptotic bodies, fragmented DNA, and arrest in the sub-G1 cell cycle phase. Alterations in mitochondrial membrane potential and the increased production of ROS were also observed (Faheina-Martins et al., 2012).

ConA is therefore considered a potential antineoplastic agent and has already been tested in preclinical or clinical trials for cancer therapeutics (Annabi et al., 2016) owing to its ability to induce both autophagy and apoptosis in several cancer cell lines.

The mistletoe lectins have been used in Europe as alternative adjuvant agent in cancer therapy, reducing the adverse effects of chemo- and radiotherapies, and improving the patient's quality of life (Schumacher et al., 2003). Strategies to improve the delivery method of mistletoe lectins have been studied and it has been suggested that enteric-coated mistletoe treatment might play an important role in the inhibition of tumor progression in murine melanoma *in vivo* (Han et al., 2015).

Viscum album (European mistletoe) agglutinins (VAA-I, II, and III) are three different proteins that have been isolated from leaves and possess different carbohydrate specificities: VAA-I has a high affinity for D-galactose, VAA-III for *N*-acetyl-galactosamine, and VAA-II for both sugars (Franz, 1986). They belong to the class of type II ribosome-inactivating proteins (RIPs). Among them, VAA-I is the most studied and consists of an A chain that inactivates the 60S ribosomal subunit and a B chain capable of binding to cell-surface glycoconjugates (Ye et al., 2006). Cytotoxic effects were induced by all VAAs on sensitive (HT 29mdr−) and multidrug-resistant (HT 29mdr+) human colon cancer cell lines *in vitro* (Valentiner et al., 2002). VAA also dose-dependently induced apoptosis in human lymphoblastic leukemia cells (NALM-6) (Seifert et al., 2008). *V. album* leaves contain triterpene acids, which are able to embed in membranes and disturb their structure, thereby facilitating the migration of VAA into the cytoplasm and enhancing the therapeutic value of this lectin (Mulsow et al., 2016).

V. album var. *coloratum* (Korean mistletoe) agglutinin (VCA) is a lectin isolated from extract of *leaves* and stems (Park et al., 1997) that shows sugar specificity for D-galactose and *N*-acetylgalactosamine (Lyu et al., 2000). VCA induced strong G0/G1 cell cycle arrest and apoptosis in murine melanoma cells (B16BL6 and B16F10) and regulation of the expression of multiple caspases was observed (Han et al., 2015). The remarkable antineoplastic activity of VCA towards colorectal cancers cells (HT-29 and CLY cell lines) has been demonstrated *in vitro* and *in vivo* (Li et al., 2011b) and the induction of apoptosis in human hepatocarcinoma cells (SK-Hep-1 and Hep 3B) was shown to be associated with inhibition of telomerase, the downregulation of Bcl-2, and the upregulation of Bax functioning upstream of caspase-3 (Lyu et al., 2002). The combination of VCA and DOX resulted in a strong synergistic effect in human breast cancer cells (MCF-7 and MDA-MB231), with growth inhibition, the stimulation of proteins such as Bax, and the inhibition of Bcl-2 (Wang et al., 2010).

Polygonatum cyrtonema lectin (PCL), a member of the *Galanthus nivalis* agglutinin (GNA) family, is a mannose and sialic acid-binding lectin isolated from rhizomes (An et al., 2006). Many studies of PCL have revealed interesting results, such as antineoplastic activities in MCF-7, A375 and mouse fibrosarcoma (L929) cells. PCL can induce apoptosis in MCF-7 and L929 cells through a caspase-dependent pathway (Liu et al., 2009b; Zhang et al., 2010). In A375 cells, PCL induced both apoptosis and autophagy via the mitochondrially-mediated ROS-p38-p53 pathway. The mechanism of apoptosis after treatment with PCL also involved the upregulation of Bax protein and the downregulation of Bcl-2 and Bcl-xL. Treatment with PCL abrogated the glutathione antioxidant system and induced massive ROS accumulation in mitochondria (Liu et al., 2009a).

POL is a mannose-binding lectin purified from the rhizomes of another *Polygonatum* species (*P. odoratum*). It is a homotetramer composed of four 11.9 kDa subunits and is also categorized as part of the GNA-related family a group of lectins (Yang et al., 2011). It showed remarkable effects on the growth of A375 cells (IC_{50} = 25 μg/mL) through the induction of apoptosis via a caspase-dependent mechanism (Yang et al., 2011). POL exerted antiproliferative effect on L929 growth (IC_{50} = 25 μg/mL), inducing apoptosis in a caspase-dependent manner through both the mitochondrial and death-receptor pathways (Fas-mediated and TNF-α) (Liu et al., 2009c). This lectin also induced apoptosis in non-small cell lung carcinoma (A549 cells; IC_{50} = 23 μg/mL) by triggering apoptosis through the suppression of the Akt-NF-κB pathways and by initiating autophagy via the inhibition of the Akt-mTOR pathway; the activation of caspases 3 and 9, the release of cytochrome c, the reduction of mitochondrial membrane potential, the upregulation of Bax and Bid, the downregulation of Bcl-2, Bcl-X, and ROS production (Li et al., 2014) were observed. More recently, it was shown that the induction of apoptosis and autophagy in A549 cells by POL was linked to regulation of microRNA-1290 and microRNA-15a-3p (Wu et al., 2016). Other study showed that POL induced apoptosis and autophagy in MCF-7 cells by targeting the ERK signaling pathway (Ouyang et al., 2014).

The *Ricinus communis* seed lectin (ricin), the first described lectin, is composed of two different polypeptide chains of approximately 30–35 kDa. Each is formed by the toxin ricin, an A-chain which blocks polypeptide chain elongation in eukaryotic cell-free systems, and a nontoxic agglutinin, a B-chain that binds to galactose or *N*-acetylgalactosamine (Olsnes and Pihl, 1973). The ricin B-chain binds to cell surface receptors containing galactose or *N*-acetylgalactosamine and facilitates the internalization of ricin A-chain into cells by receptor mediated endocytosis, causing leading to cell death (Wales et al., 1992; Lord et al., 2003). Despite its toxic effects, ricin is considered to have potential benefits in the treatment of a variety of cancers, including leukemia, breast cancer, cervical cancer, and melanoma (Tyagi et al., 2013; Tyagi et al., 2015).

Ricin A-chain has RNA *N*-glycosidase activity, which inactivates eukaryotic ribosomes (Endo and Tsurugi, 1987) and conjugates of ricin A-chain with antibodies against cancer cells, has been developed as a therapeutic agent (Weidle et al., 2014). The results of a randomized phase III study in 157 patients with B-cell lymphoma showed that ricin therapy tended to improve survival, although no significant differences were found in event-free survival and overall survival compared with the control (Furman et al., 2011). Ricin B-chain may be an efficient vehicle for the generation of cell-mediated immune responses and this chain may also increase the therapeutic potential of protein-based vaccines against cervical cancer in women (Sadraeian et al., 2013). In its integral form and at very low concentrations, ricin showed the potential to decrease the size of tumors formed in soft agar and increase apoptosis of human malignant melanoma cells (SKMEL28) via downregulation of ERK signaling. These results suggested that ricin can be used as a drug for melanoma treatment (Trung et al., 2016).

However, several side effects discontinue the clinical trials of ricin. Ricin B-chain can bind to glycoproteins and glycolipids present on the surface of almost every kind of cells, which limits the potential application of ricin as an anticancer agent (Audi et al., 2005). Thus, the use of ricin still requires further study.

Table 1. Plant lectins with antineoplastic activity and mechanisms of cytotoxic action

Plant source	Abbreviation	Cancer cell or model	Mechanism involved	Reference
Abelmoschus esculentus (seeds)	AEL	MCF-7	Apoptosis, increase of Bax/Bcl-2 ratio increased, activation of caspase-3 and -9	Monte et al. (2014)
Artocarpus heterophyllus (seeds)	Jacalin	H1299, MCF-7	Cell growth inhibition	Zuraidah et al. (2014)
Astragalus membranaceus (roots)	AML	K562	Apoptosis caspase-dependent mechanism, and decreased Bcl-2	Huang et al. (2012)
		HeLa	Cell growth inhibition	Yan et al. (2010)
Bauhinia ungulata (seeds)	BUL	HT-29	Cell growth inhibition	Silva et al. (2014a)
Bauhinia forficata (seeds)	BfL	MCF-7	Inhibition of cell growth, DNA fragmentation, cycle arrest in G2/M and inhibits adhesion, cell death with inhibition of caspase-9. Death by necrosis	Silva et al. (2014b)
Benincasa hispida (fruit)	BhL	A549, HeLa, PANC-1, CFPAC-1, MIA PaCa-2	Cell growth inhibition. Apoptosis with caspase-9 and -3 activations in PANC-1, CFPAC-1 and MIA PaCa-2.	Singh et al. (2016)
Canavalia brasiliensis (seeds)	ConBr	MOLT4, HL-60	Apoptosis/necrosis, mitochondrial depolarization, increase in ROS production	Faheina-Martins et al., (2012)
Canavalia virosa (seeds)	ConV	C6	Cytoxicity, induced autophagy, decreased mitochondrial membrane potential	Osterne et al. (2017)
Calliandra surinamensis (leaf)	CasuL	K562, T47D	Cell growth inhibition	Procópio et al. (2017)
Cratylia mollis (seeds)	Cramoll	PC-3	Cell growth inhibition, loss of membrane integrity, increase cytosolic calcium and mitochondrial superoxide anion	Andrade et al. (2004)
	rCramoll	PC-3	Lose of membrane integrity, increase of cytosolic calcium and mitochondrial superoxide anion levels	Figueirôa et al. (2017)
		Sarcoma 180	Tumor growth inhibition	Cunha et al. (2016)

Plant source	Abbreviation	Cancer cell or model	Mechanism involved	Reference
Datura innoxia (seeds)	DiL9	A549, HeLa, PANC-1, CFPAC-1, MIA PaCa-2	Cell growth inhibition. Apoptosis with caspase-9 and -3 activations in PANC-1, CFPAC-1 and MIA PaCa-2	Singh et al. (2016)
Dioscorea opposite (tubers)	----	MCF-7, HepG2, CNE2	Cell growth inhibition, Apoptosis, mitochondrial depolarization	Chan and Ng (2013)
Euphorbia tirucalli (latex)	Eutirucallin	HeLa, PC3, MDA-MB-231, MCF-7	Antiproliferative activity	Palharini et al. (2017)
		Ehrlich ascites carcinoma	Inhibition of carcinoma in vivo	Palharini et al. (2017)
Lotus corniculatus (seeds)	LCL	THP-1, HOP62, HCT116	Cell growth inhibition, apoptosis, increased sub G0/G1 ratio, mitochondrial depolarization	Rafiq et al. (2013)
Moringa oleifera (seeds)	MOSL	Ehrlich ascites carcinoma	Cell growth inhibition, cell cycle arrest (G2/M phase), induction of apoptosis through caspase-3 dependent pathway and inhibition of NFkB signaling pathway	Asaduzzaman et al. (2018)
	cMoL	B16-F10	Induction of necrosis and apoptosis in a caspase-dependent manner (promoted activation of caspases 3, 8 and 9), increased the production of mitochondrial reactive oxygen species	Luz et al. (2017)
Morus alba (leaf)	MLL	MCF-7, HCT15	Apoptosis, up-regulation of caspase 3 activity	Deepa et al. (2012)
Pinellia ternata (Bulbs)	PTL	HeLa, K562	Cell growth inhibition	Zuo et al. (2012)
		Sarcoma 180	Inhibition of cell growth due to the arrest of DNA replication in the cell cycle (G1/S transitions)	Zuo et al. (2012)
Phaseolus vulgaris (seeds)	PHA	MCF-7, HepG2, CNE1, CNE2	Cell growth inhibition	Chan et al. (2012)
Sophora alopecuroides (seeds)	SAL	HeLa	Cell growth inhibition	Li et al. (2012)

Table 1. (Continued)

Plant source	Abbreviation	Cancer cell or model	Mechanism involved	Reference
Sophora flavescens (rhizomes)	SFL	HeLa	Caspase-dependent apoptosis	Liu et al. (2008)
Glycine max (seeds)	SBL	HeLa	Apoptosis and autophagy mediated by ROS, caspase-dependent activation	Panda et al. (2014)

A549: human pulmonary adenocarcinoma; B16F10: murine melanoma cells; CFPAC-1: human pancreatic adenocarcinoma; CNE1: human nasopharyngeal carcinoma; CNE2: human nasopharyngeal carcinoma drug-resistant; C6: rat glioma cells; H1299: human non-small *cell* lung carcinoma; HCT116: human colon cancer; HCT15: human colon cancer; HeLa: human cervical cancer; HepG2: human hepatoma; HL-60: human promyelocytic leukemia; HOP62: human lung cancer; HT-29: human colon adenocarcinoma; *K562: human chronic myeloid leukemia*; MCF7: human breast carcinoma; MDAMB-231: human breast cancer; MIA PaCa-2: human pancreatic cancer; MOLT4: human acute lymphoblastic leukemia; PANC 1: human pancreatic carcinoma; PC-3: human prostate cancer; T47D: human breast tumor; THP-1: human acute monocytic leukemia.

In addition to these lectins commented above, experiments have been conducted to investigate the cytotoxicity and action mechanisms of several other plant lectins in human cancer cell lines. Other plant lectins with anticancer effects are presented in Table 1.

CONCLUSION

As conventional cancer chemotherapy may have severe side effects in patients with cancer, the demand for alternative treatments is constant. Plant lectins have been studied widely as possible alternatives for new chemotherapeutics and, in this paper, we have provided an overview of their potential. Studies of the action mechanisms of plant lectins have reported that their antineoplastic activity may be linked to interaction with specific receptors on the cell membrane or internalization via endocytosis. In both cases, the lectins can cause cell growth inhibition and/or death by several mechanisms: the inhibition of cell growth and survival pathways, cell cycle arrest, induction of oxidative stress, activation of apoptosis (via the intrinsic and extrinsic pathways), and the stimulation of autophagy. Some lectins have been studied in clinical trials, but there are many lectins with reported *in vitro* anticancer properties that deserves further evaluation of their potential for development as anticancer drugs. Finally, as a plant lectin often acts on cancer cells through multiple targets, this may help prevent the development of chemotherapeutic resistance. In addition, these classes of proteins are usually less toxic to normal cells than the current drug options.

Acknowledgments

The authors express their gratitude to the *Conselho Nacional de Desenvolvimento Científico e Tecnológico* (CNPq) for research grants and fellowship (PMGP and THN) as well as to the *Fundação de Amparo à Ciência e Tecnologia do Estado de Pernambuco* (FACEPE; APQ-0108-2.08/14) for financial support and graduate scholarship (IBPG-1712-2.08/16).

References

Al-Mamun, M. A., Akter, Z., Uddin, M. J., Ferdaus, K. M. K. B., Hoque, K. M. F., Ferdousi, Z., Reza, M. A. (2016). Characterization and evaluation of antibacterial and antiproliferative activities of crude protein extracts isolated from the seed of *Ricinus communis* in Bangladesh. *BMC Complement. Altern. Med.* 16: 211-221.

Ambasta, R. K., Jha, S. K., Kumar, D., Sharma, R., Jha, N. K., Kumar, P. (2015). Comparative study of anti-angiogenic activities of luteolin, lectin and lupeol biomolecules. *J. Transl. Med.* 13: 307-316.

Amin, A. R. M. R., Paul, R. K., Thakur, V. S., Agarwal, M. L. (2007). A novel role for p73 in the regulation of Akt-Foxo1a-Bim signaling and apoptosis induced by the plant lectin, concanavalin A. *Cancer Res.* 67: 5617-5621.

An, J., Liu, J. Z., Wu, C. F., Li, J., Dai, L., Van Damme, E., Balzarini, J., De Clercq, E., Chen, F., Bao, J. K. (2006). Anti-HIV I/II activity and molecular cloning of a novel mannose/sialic acid-binding lectin from rhizome of *Polygonatum cyrtonema* Hua. *Acta Biochim. Biophys. Sin.* 38: 70-78.

Andrade, C. A. S., Correia, M. T. S., Coelho, L. C. B. B., Nascimento, S. C., Santos-Magalhães, N. S. (2004). Antitumor activity of *Cratylia mollis* lectin encapsulated into liposomes. *Int. J. Pharm.* 278: 435-445.

Annabi, B., Burke Nanni, S., Pratt, J., Beauchemin, D., Haidara, K., Annabi, B. (2016). Impact of concanavalin-a-mediated cytoskeleton disruption on low-density lipoprotein receptor-related protein-1 internalization and cell surface expression in glioblastomas. *Biomark. Cancer* 8: 77-87.

Arul, D., Subramanian, P. (2013). Naringenin (*Citrus flavonone*) induces growth inhibition, cell cycle arrest and apoptosis in human hepatocellular carcinoma cells. *Pathol. Oncol. Res.* 19: 763-70.

Asaduzzaman, A. K. M., Hasan, I., Chakrabortty, A., Zaman, S., Islam, S. S., Ahmed, F. R. S., Kabir, K. M. A., Nurujjaman, M., Uddin, M. B., Alam, M. T., Shaha, R. K., Kabir, S. R. (2018). *Moringa oleifera* seed lectin inhibits Ehrlich ascites carcinoma cell growth by inducing apoptosis through the regulation of Bak and NF-κB gene expression. *Int. J. Biol. Macromol.* 107: 1936-1944.

Audi, J., Belson, M., Patel, M., Schier, J., Osterloh, J. (2005). Ricin poisoning: A comprehensive review. *JAMA* 294: 2342-2351.

Aunan, J. R., Cho, W. C., Søreide, K. (2017). The biology of aging and cancer: a brief overview of shared and divergent molecular hallmarks. *Aging Dis.* 8: 1-15.

Bagaria, A., Surendranath, K., Ramagopal, U. A., Ramakumar, S., Karande, A. A. (2006). Structure-function analysis and insights into the reduced toxicity of *Abrus precatorius* agglutinin I in relation to abrin. *J. Biol. Chem.* 281: 34465-34474.

Bhutia, S. K., Behera, B., Nandini Das, D., Mukhopadhyay, S., Sinha, N., Panda, P. K., Naik, P. P., Patra, S. K., Mandal, M., Sarkar, S., Menezes, M. E., Talukdar, S., Maiti, T. K., Das, S. K., Sarkar, D., Fisher, P.B.

(2016). Abrus agglutinin is a potent anti-proliferative and anti-Angiogenic agent in human breast cancer. *Int. J. Cancer* 139: 457-466.

Bhutia, S. K., Mallick, S. K., Maiti, S., Maiti, T. K. (2009a). Inhibitory effect of *Abrus* abrin-derived peptide fraction against Dalton's lymphoma ascites model. *Phytomedicine* 16: 377–385.

Bhutia, S. K., Mallick, S. K., Maiti, S., Mishra, D., Maiti, T. K. (2009b). *Abrus* abrin derived peptides induce apoptosis by targeting mitochondria in HeLa cells. *Cell Biol. Int.* 33: 720-727.

Blériot, C., Lecuit, M. (2016). The interplay between regulated necrosis and bacterial infection. *Cell. Mol. Life Sci.* 73: 2369-2378.

Campos, J. K. L., Araújo, C. S. F., Araújo, T. F. S., Santos, A. F. S., Teixeira, J. A., Lima, V. L. M., Coelho, L. C. B. B. (2016). Anti-inflammatory and antinociceptive activities of *Bauhinia monandra* leaf lectin. *Biochimie Open* 2: 62-68.

Chan, Y. S., Ng, T. B. (2013b). A lectin with highly potent inhibitory activity toward breast cancer cells from edible tubers of *Dioscorea opposita* cv. Nagaimo. *PLoS One* 8: e54212.

Chan, Y. S., Wong, J. H., Fang, E. F., Pan, W., Ng, T. B. (2012). Isolation of a glucosamine binding leguminous lectin with mitogenic activity towards splenocytes and anti-proliferative activity towards tumor cells. *PLoS One* 7: e3896.

Chang, C. P., Yang, M. C., Liu, H. S., Lin, Y. S., Lei, H. Y. (2007). Concanavalin A induces autophagy in hepatoma cells and has a therapeutic effect in a murine in situ hepatoma model. *Hepatology* 45: 286-296.

Choi, A. M. K., Ryter, S. W., Levine, B. (2013). Autophagy in human health and disease. *N. Engl. J. Med.* 368: 651-662.

Christiansen, M. N., Chik, J., Lee, L., Anugraham, M., Abrahams, J. L., Packer, N. H. (2014). Cell surface protein glycosylation in cancer. *Proteomics* 14: 525-546.

Ciomber, A., Smagur, A., Mitrus, I., Cichoń, T., Smolarczyk, R., Sochanik, A., Szala, S., Jarosz, M. (2013). Antitumor effects of recombinant antivascular protein ABRaA-VEGF121 combined with IL-12 gene therapy. *Arch. Immunol. Ther. Exp.* 62: 161-168.

Cunha, C. R. A., Silva, L. C. N., Almeida, F. J. F., Ferraz, M. S., Varejão, N., Cartaxo, M. F. S., de Miranda, R. C. M., Aguiar, F. C. A., Santos, N.P.S., Coelho, L. C. B. B., Santos-Magalhães, N. S., Correia, M. T. S. (2016). Encapsulation into stealth liposomes enhances the antitumor action of recombinant *Cratylia mollis* lectin expressed in *Escherichia coli*. *Front. Microbiol.* 7: 1355.

Deepa, M., Sureshkumar, T., Satheeshkumar, P. K., Priya, S. (2012). Purified mulberry leaf lectin (MLL) induces apoptosis and cell cycle arrest in human breast cancer and colon cancer cells. *Chem. Biol. Interact.* 200: 38-44.

Derbal, Y. (2017). Perspective on the dynamics of cancer. *Theor. Biol. Med. Model.* 14: 1-18.

Dhanasekaran, R., Kwo, P. Y. (2017). The liver in Oncology. *Clin. Liver Dis.* 21: 697-707.

Dias, R. O., Santos Machado, L., Migliolo, L., Franco, O. L. (2015). Insights into animal and plant lectins with antimicrobial activities. *Molecules* 20: 519-541.

Dickson, M. A., Schwartz, G. K. (2009). Development of cell-cycle inhibitors for cancer therapy. *Curr. Oncol.* 16: 36-43.

Endo, Y., Tsurugi, K. (1987). RNA N-glycosidase activity of ricin A-chain. Mechanism of action of the toxic lectin ricin on eukaryotic ribosomes. *J. Biol. Chem.* 262: 8128-8130.

Estrada-Martínez, L. E., Moreno-Celis, U., Cervantes-Jiménez, R., Ferriz-Martínez, R. A., Blanco-Labra, A., García-Gasca, T. (2017). Plant lectins as medical tools against digestive system cancers. *Int. J. Mol. Sci.* 18: 1403-1421.

Faheina-Martins, G. V., da Silveira, A. L., Cavalcanti, B. C., Ramos, M. V., Moraes, M. O., Pessoa, C., Araújo, D. A. M. (2012). Antiproliferative effects of lectins from *Canavalia ensiformis* and *Canavalia brasiliensis* in human leukemia cell lines. *Toxicol. in Vitro* 26: 1161-1169.

Faraji, A., Manshadi, H. R. D., Mobaraki, M., Zare, M., Houshmand, M. (2016). Association of ABCB1 and SLC22A16 gene polymorphisms with incidence of doxorubicin-induced febrile neutropenia: A survey of iranian breast cancer patients. *PLoS One* 11: e0168519.

Ferlay, J., Soerjomataram, I., Dikshit, R., Eser, S., Mathers, C., Rebelo, M., Parkin, D.M., Forman, D., Bray, F. (2015). Cancer incidence and mortality worldwide: Sources, methods and major patterns in GLOBOCAN 2012. *Int. J. Cancer* 136: E359-E386.

Figueirôa, E. O., Aranda-Souza, M. Â., Varejão, N., Rossato, F. A., Costa, R. A. P., Figueira, T. R., Silva, L. C. N., Castilho, R. F., Vercesi, A. E., Correia, M. T. S. (2017). pCramoll and rCramoll lectins induce cell death in human prostate adenocarcinoma (PC-3) cells by impairment of mitochondrial homeostasis. *Toxicol. Vitr.* 43: 40-46.

Franz, H. (1986). Mistletoe lectins and their A and B chains. *Oncology* 43: 23-34.

Furman, R. R., Grossbard, M. L., Johnson, J. L., Pecora, A. L., Cassileth, P. A., Jung, S. H., Peterson, B. A., Nadler, L. M., Freedman, A., Bayer, R. L., Bartlett, N. L., Hurd, D. D., Cheson, B. D. (2011). A phase III study of anti-B4-blocked ricin as adjuvant therapy post-autologous bone marrow transplant: CALGB 9254. *Leuk Lymphoma* 52: 587-596.

Gabor, F., Klausegger, U., Wirth, M. (2001). The interaction between wheat germ agglutinin and other plant lectins with prostate cancer cells Du-145. *Int. J. Pharm.* 221: 35-47.

Ghazarian, H., Idoni, B., Oppenheimer, S. B. (2011). A glycobiology review: carbohydrates, lectins and implications in cancer therapeutics. *Acta Histochem.* 113: 236-247.

Ghosh, D., Maiti, T. K. (2007). Immunomodulatory and anti-tumor activities of native and heat denatured *Abrus* agglutinin. *Immunobiology* 212: 589-599.

Hamid, R., Masood, A., Wani, I. H., Rafiq, S. (2013). Lectins: Proteins with diverse applications. *J. Appl. Pharm. Sci.* 3: 93-103.

Han, S. Y., Hong, C. E., Kim, H. G., Lyu, S. Y. (2015). Anti-cancer effects of enteric-coated polymers containing mistletoe lectin in murine melanoma cells in vitro and in vivo. *Mol. Cell. Biochem.* 408: 14-16.

Hata, A. N., Engelman, J. A., Faber, A. C. (2015). The BCL2 family: Key mediators of the apoptotic response to targeted anticancer therapeutics. *Cancer Discov.* 5: 475-487.

Huang, L. H., Yan, Q. J., Kopparapu, N. K., Jiang, Z. Q., Sun, Y. (2012). *Astragalus membranaceus* lectin (AML) induces caspase-dependent apoptosis in human leukemia cells. *Cell Prolif.* 45: 15-21.

Kepp, O., Galluzzi, L., Lipinski, M., Yuan, J., Kroemer, G. (2011). Cell death assays for drug discovery. *Nat. Rev. Drug Discov.* 10: 221-237.

Kumar, V., Abbas, A. K., Fausto, N., Mitchell, R. N. (2007). Robbins Basic Pathology, eighth edition, Saunders/Elsevier.

Li, C., Chen, J., Lu, B., Shi, Z., Wang, H., Zhang, B., Zhao, K., Qi, W., Bao, J., Wang, Y. (2014). Molecular switch role of Akt in *Polygonatum odoratum* lectin-induced apoptosis and autophagy in human non-small cell lung cancer A549 cells. *PLoS One* 9: e101526.

Li, L. N., Zhang, H. D., Zhi, R., Yuan, S. J. (2011b). Down-regulation of some miRNAs by degrading their precursors contributes to anti-cancer effect of mistletoe lectin-I. *Br. J. Pharmacol.* 162: 349-364.

Li, T., Yin, X., Liu, D., Ma, X., Lv, H., Sun, S. (2012). Isolation and characterization of a novel lectin with antifungal and antiproliferative activities from *Sophora alopecuroides* seeds. *Acta Biochim. Biophys. Sin.* 44: 606-613.

Li, W. W., Yu, J Y., Xu, H. L., Bao, J. K. (2011a). Concanavalin A: A potential anti-neoplastic agent targeting apoptosis, autophagy and anti-angiogenesis for cancer therapeutics. *Biochem. Biophys. Res. Commun.* 414: 282-286.

Lima, T. A., Fernandes, K. M., Oliveira, A. P. S., Dornelles, L. P., Martins, G. F., Napoleão, T. H., Paiva, P. M. (2017). Termiticidal lectins from *Myracrodruon urundeuva* (Anacardiaceae) cause midgut damage when ingested by *Nasutitermes corniger* (Isoptera: Termitidae) workers. *Pest Manag. Sci.* 73: 991-998.

Liu, B., Bian, H. jiao, Bao, J. (2010). Plant lectins: potential antineoplastic drugs from bench to clinic. *Cancer Lett.* 287: 1-12.

Liu, B., Cheng, Y., Bian, H. J., Bao, J. K. (2009a). Molecular mechanisms of *Polygonatum cyrtonema* lectin-induced apoptosis and autophagy in cancer cells. *Autophagy* 5: 253-255.

Liu, B., Li, C. Y., Bian, H. J., Min, M. W., Chen, L. F., Bao, J. K. (2009d). Antiproliferative activity and apoptosis-inducing mechanism of

Concanavalin A on human melanoma A375 cells, *Arch. Biochem. Biophys.* 482: 1–6.

Liu, B., Peng, H., Yao, Q., Li, J., Damme, E. Van, Balzarini, J. (2009b). Bioinformatics analyses of the mannose-binding lectins from *Polygonatum cyrtonema*, *Ophiopogon japonicus* and *Liparis noversa* with antiproliferative and apoptosis-inducing activities. *Phytomedicine* 16: 601–608.

Liu, B., Zhang, B., Min, M. wei, Bian, H. jiao, Chen, L. fei, Liu, Q., Bao, J. (2009c). Induction of apoptosis by *Polygonatum odoratum* lectin and its molecular mechanisms in murine fibrosarcoma L929 cells. *Biochim. Biophys. Acta - Gen. Subj.* 1790: 840-844.

Liu, C. L., Tsai, C. C., Lin, S. C., Wang, L. I., Hsu, C. I., Hwang, M. J., Lin, J. Y. (2000). Primary structure and function analysis of the *Abrus precatorius* agglutinin A chain by site-directed mutagenesis. Pro199 of amphiphilic α-helix h impairs protein synthesis inhibitory activity. *J. Biol. Chem.* 275: 1897-1901.

Liu, Z., Liu, B., Zhang, Z., Zhou, T., Bian, H., Min, M., Liu, Y., Chen, J., Bao, J. (2008). A mannose-binding lectin from *Sophora flavescens* induces apoptosis in HeLa cells. *Phytomedicine* 15: 867-875.

LoPiccolo, J., Blumenthal, G. M., Bernstein, W. B., Dennis, P. A. (2008). Targeting the PI3K/Akt/mTOR pathway: Effective combinations and clinical considerations. *Drug Resist. Updat.* 11: 32-50.

Lord, M. J., Jolliffe, N. A., Marsden, C. J., Pateman, C. S. C., Smith, D. C., Spooner, R. A., Watson, P. D., Roberts, L.M. (2003). Ricin: mechanisms of cytotoxicity. *Toxicol.* Rev. 22: 53-64.

Luz, L. A., Rossato, F. A., Costa, R. A. P., Napoleão, T. H., Paiva, P. M. G., Coelho, L. C. B. B. (2017). Cytotoxicity of the coagulant *Moringa oleifera* lectin (cMoL) to B16-F10 melanoma cells. *Toxicol. in Vitro* 44: 94-99.

Lyu, S. Y., Choi, S. H., Park, W. B. (2002). Korean mistletoe lectin-induced apoptosis in hepatocarcinoma cells is associated with inhibition of telomerase via mitochondrial controlled pathway independent of p53. *Arch. Pharm. Res.* 25: 93-101.

Lyu, S. Y., Park, S. M., Choung, B. Y., Park, W. B. (2000). Comparative study of Korean (*Viscum album* var. *coloratum*) and European mistletoes (*Viscum album*). *Arch. Pharm. Res.* 23: 592-598.

Matallanas, D., Birtwistle, M., Romano, D., Zebisch, A., Rauch, J., von Kriegsheim, A., Kolch, W. (2011). Raf family kinases: old dogs have learned new tricks. *Genes Cancer* 2: 232-260.

McIlwain, D. R., Berger, T., Mak, T. W. (2013). Caspase Functions in Cell Death and Disease. *Cold Spring Harb. Perspect. Biol.* 5: a008656-a008656.

Mehrzadi, S., Fatemi, I., Esmaeilizadeh, M., Ghaznavi, H., Kalantar, H., Goudarzi, M. (2018). Hepatoprotective effect of berberine against methotrexate induced liver toxicity in rats. *Biomed. Pharmacother.* 97: 233-239.

Mejía, E. G., Prisecaru, V. I. (2005). Lectins as bioactive plant proteins: a potential in cancer treatment. *Crit. Rev. Food Sci. Nutr.* 45: 425-445.

Monte, L. G., Santi-Gadelha, T., Reis, L. B., Braganhol, E., Prietsch, R. F., Dellagostin, O. A., Lacerda, R. R., Gadelha, C. A. A., Conceição, F. R., Pinto, L. S. (2014). Lectin of *Abelmoschus esculentus* (okra) promotes selective antitumor effects in human breast cancer cells. *Biotechnol. Lett.* 36: 461-469.

Moura, M. C., Napoleão, T. H., Coriolano, M. C., Paiva, P. M. G., Figueiredo, R. C. B. Q., Coelho, L. C. B. B. (2015). Water-soluble *Moringa oleifera* lectin interferes with growth, survival and cell permeability of corrosive and pathogenic bacteria. *J. Appl. Microbiol.* 119: 666-676.

Mukhopadhyay, S., Panda, P. K., Das, D. N., Sinha, N., Behera, B., Maiti, T. K., Bhutia, S. K. (2014). *Abrus* agglutinin suppresses human hepatocellular carcinoma in vitro and in vivo by inducing caspase-mediated cell death. *Acta Pharmacol.* Sin. 35: 814-824.

Mulsow, K., Enzlein, T., Delebinski, C., Jaeger, S., Seifert, G., Melzig, M. F. (2016). Impact of mistletoe triterpene acids on the uptake of mistletoe lectin by cultured tumor cells. *PLoS One* 11: e0153825.

Narayanan, S., Surolia, A., Karande, A. A. (2004). Ribosome-inactivating protein and apoptosis: abrin causes cell death via mitochondrial pathway in Jurkat cells. *Biochem. J.* 377: 233-240.

Olsnes, S., Pihl, A. (1973). Different biological properties of the two constituent peptide chains of ricin, a toxic protein inhibiting protein synthesis. *Biochemistry* 12: 3121-3126.

Osterne, V. J. S., Silva-Filho, J. C., Santiago, M. Q., Pinto-Junior, V. R., Almeida, A. C., Barreto, A. A. G. C., Wolin, I.A.V., Nascimento, A. P. M., Amorim, R. M. F., Rocha, B.A.M., Delatorre, P., Nagano, C. S., Leal, R. B., Assreuy, A. M. S., Nascimento, K. S., Cavada, B. S. (2017). Structural characterization of a lectin from *Canavalia virosa* seeds with inflammatory and cytotoxic activities. *Int. J. Biol. Macromol.* 94: 271-282.

Otto, T., Sicinski, P. (2017). Cell cycle proteins as promising targets in cancer therapy. *Nat. Rev. Cancer* 17: 93-115.

Ouyang, L., Chen, Y., Wang, X. Y., Lu, R. F., Zhang, S. Y., Tian, M., Xie, T., Liu, B., He, G. (2014). *Polygonatum odoratum* lectin induces apoptosis and autophagy via targeting EGFR-mediated Ras-Raf-MEK-ERK pathway in human MCF-7 breast cancer cells. *Phytomedicine* 21: 1658-1665.

Paiva, P. M. G., Napoleão, T. H., Santos, N. D. L., Correia, M. T. S., Navarro, D. M. A. F., Coelho, L. C. B. B. (2011). Plant compounds with *Aedes Aegypti* larvicidal activity and other biological properties. In: Liong, M. T. (Ed.), Bioprocess Sciences and Technology, Nova Science Publishers Inc. New York, pp. 271-296.

Palharini, J. G., Richter, A. C., Silva, M. F., Ferreira, F. B., Pirovani, C. P., Naves, K. S. C., Goulart, V. A., Mineo, T. W. P., Silva, M. J. B., Santiago, F. M. (2017). Eutirucallin: A Lectin with Antitumor and Antimicrobial Properties. *Front. Cell. Infect. Microbiol.* 7, 1-13.

Pan, S. T., Li, Z. L., He, Z. X., Qiu, J. X., Zhou, S. F. (2016). Molecular mechanisms for tumour resistance to chemotherapy. *Clin. Exp. Pharmacol. Physiol.* 43: 723-737.

Panda, P. K., Mukhopadhyay, S., Behera, B., Bhol, C. S., Dey, S., Das, D. N., Sinha, N., Bissoyi, A., Pramanik, K., Maiti, T. K., Bhutia, S. K.

(2014). Antitumor effect of soybean lectin mediated through reactive oxygen species-dependent pathway. *Life Sci.* 111: 27-35.

Park, W. B., Han, S. K., Lee, M. H., Han, K. H. (1997). Isolation and characterization of lectins from stem and leaves of Korean mistletoe (*Viscum album* var. *coloratum*) by affinity chromatography. *Arch. Pharm. Res.* 20: 306-312.

Parrales, A., Iwakuma, T. (2015). Targeting oncogenic mutant p53 for cancer therapy. *Front. Oncol.* 5: 1-13.

Parrish, A. B., Freel, C. D., Kornbluth, S. (2013). Cellular mechanisms controlling caspase activation and function. *Cold Spring Harb. Perspect. Biol.* 5: a008672-a008672.

Patriota, L. L. S., Procópio, T. F., Brito, J. S., Sebag, V., Oliveira, A. P. S., Soares, A. K. A., Moreira, L. R., Lima, T. A., Soares, T., Silva, T. D., Paiva, P. M. G., Lorena, V. M. B., Melo, C. M. L., Albuquerque, L. P., Napoleão, T. H. (2017). *Microgramma vacciniifolia* (Polypodiaceae) fronds contain a multifunctional lectin with immunomodulatory properties on human cells. *Int. J. Biol. Macromol.* 103: 36-46.

Porta, C., Paglino, C., Mosca, A. (2014). Targeting PI3K/Akt/mTOR signaling in cancer. *Front. Oncol.* 4: 64.

Powathil, G. G., Chaplain, M. A. J., Swat, M. (2014). Investigating the development of chemotherapeutic drug resistance in cancer: A multiscale computational study. arXiv:1407.0865.

Pratt, J., Annabi, B. (2014). Induction of autophagy biomarker BNIP3 requires a JAK2/STAT3 and MT1-MMP signaling interplay in Concanavalin-A-activated U87 glioblastoma cells. *Cell. Signal.* 26: 917-924.

Pratt, J., Roy, R., Annabi, B. (2012). Concanavalin-A-induced autophagy biomarkers requires membrane type-1 matrix metalloproteinase intracellular signaling in glioblastoma cells. *Glycobiology* 22: 1245-1255.

Procópio, T. F., Patriota, L L. S., Moura, M. C., Silva, P. M., Oliveira, A. P. S., Carvalho, L. V. N., Lima, T. A., Soares, T., Silva, T. D., Coelho, L. C. B. B., Pitta, M. G. R., Rêgo, M. J. B. M., Figueiredo, R. C. B. Q., Paiva, P. M. G., Napoleão, T. H. (2017). CasuL: A new lectin isolated from *Calliandra surinamensis* leaf pinnulae with cytotoxicity to cancer cells, antimicrobial activity and antibiofilm effect. *Int. J. Biol. Macromol.* 98: 419-429.

Rafiq, S., Majeed, R., Qazi, A. K., Ganai, B. A., Wani, I., Rakhshanda, S., Qurishi, Y., Sharma, P. R., Hamid, A., Masood, A., Hamid, R. (2013). Isolation and antiproliferative activity of *Lotus corniculatus* lectin towards human tumour cell lines. *Phytomedicine* 21: 30-38.

Ramnath, V., Rekha, P. S., Kuttan, G., Kuttan, R. (2009). Regulation of caspase-3 and Bcl-2 expression in daltons lymphoma ascites cells by abrin. *Evidence-Based Complement. Altern. Med.* 6: 233-238.

Reinhardt, H. C., Schumacher, B. (2012). The p53 network: cellular and systemic DNA damage responses in aging and cancer. *Trends Genet.* 28: 128-136.

Sadraeian, M., Rasoul-Amini, S., Mansoorkhani, M. J. K., Mohkam, M., Ghoshoon, M. B., Ghasemi, Y. (2013). Induction of antitumor immunity against cervical cancer by protein HPV-16 E7 in fusion with ricin B chain in tumor-bearing mice. *Int. J. Gynecol. Cancer* 23: 809-814.

Samatar, A. A., Poulikakos, P. I. (2014). Targeting RAS–ERK signalling in cancer: promises and challenges. *Nat. Rev. Drug Discov.* 13: 928-942.

Santos, A. F. S., Napoleão, T. H., Bezerra, R. F., Carvalho, E. V. M. M., Correia, M. T. S., Coelho, L. C. B. B. (2013). Strategies to obtain lectins from distinct sources In: Berhardt, L. V. (Ed.) *Advances in Medicine and Biology*, vol. 63 Nova Science Publishers Inc., New York, pp. 34-60.

Santos, P. B., Zanetti, J. S., Vieira-de-Mello, G. S., Rêgo, M. J. B. M., Ribeiro-Silva, A. A., Beltrão, E. I. C. (2014). Lectin histochemistry reveals SNA as a prognostic carbohydrate-dependent probe for invasive ductal carcinoma of the breast: A clinicopathological and immunohistochemical auxiliary tool. *Int. J. Clin. Exp. Pathol.* 7: 2337-2349.

Sato, Y., Morimoto, K., Kubo, T., Yanagihara, K., Seyama, T. (2012). High mannose-binding antiviral lectin PFL from *Pseudomonas fluorescens* Pf0-1 promotes cell death of gastric cancer cell MKN28 via interaction with α2-integrin. *PLoS One* 7: e45922.

Schumacher, K., Schneider, B., Reich, G., Stiefel, T., Stoll, G., Bock, P. R., Hanisch, J., Beuth, J. (2003). Influence of postoperative complementary treatment with lectin-standardized mistletoe extract on breast cancer patients. A controlled epidemiological multicentric retrolective cohort study. *Anticancer Res.* 23: 50810-5087.

Seifert, G., Jesse, P., Laengler, A., Reindl, T., Lüth, M., Lobitz, S., Henze, G., Prokop, A., Lode, H. N. (2008). Molecular mechanisms of mistletoe plant extract-induced apoptosis in acute lymphoblastic leukemia in vivo and in vitro. *Cancer Lett.* 264: 218-228.

Shi, Z., An, N., Zhao, S., Li, X., Bao, J. K., Yue, B. S. (2013). In silico analysis of molecular mechanisms of legume lectin-induced apoptosis in cancer cells. *Cell Prolif.* 46, 86-96.

Shi, Z., Chen, J., Li, C., An, N., Wang, Z., Yang, S., Huang, K., Bao, J. (2014). Antitumor effects of concanavalin A and *Sophora flavescens* lectin in vitro and in vivo. *Acta Pharmacol. Sin.* 35: 248-256.

Shibutani, S. T., Saitoh, T., Nowag, H., Munz, C., Yoshimori, T. (2015). Autophagy and autophagy-related proteins in the immune system. *Nat. Immunol.* 16: 1014-1024.

Silva, H. C., Pinto, L. D. S., Teixeira, E. H., Nascimento, K. S., Cavada, B. S., Silva, A. L. C. (2014a). BUL: A novel lectin from *Bauhinia ungulata* L. seeds with fungistatic and antiproliferative activities. *Process Biochem.* 49: 203-209.

Silva, M. C. C., De Paula, C. A. A., Ferreira, J. G., Paredes-Gamero, E. J., Vaz, A. M. S. F., Sampaio, M. U., Correia, M. T. S., Oliva, M. L. V. (2014b). *Bauhinia forficata* lectin (BfL) induces cell death and inhibits integrin-mediated adhesion on MCF7 human breast cancer cells. *Biochim. Biophys. Acta - Gen. Subj.* 1840: 2262-2271.

Silva, P. M., Moura, M. C., Gomes, F. S., Trentin, D. S., Oliveira, A. P. S., Melo, G. S. V., Pitta, M. G. R., Rego, M. J. B. M., Coelho, L. C. B. B., Macedo, A. J., Figueiredo, R. C. B. Q., Paiva, P. M. G., Napoleão, T. H. (2018). PgTeL, the lectin found in *Punica granatum* juice, is an antifungal agent against *Candida albicans* and *Candida krusei*. *Int. J. Biol. Macromol.* 108: 391-400.

Silva, P. M. S., Lima, A. L. R., Silva, B. V. M., Coelho, L. C. B. B., Dutra, R. F., Correia, M. T. S. (2016). *Cratylia mollis* lectin nanoelectrode for differential diagnostic of prostate cancer and benign prostatic hyperplasia based on label-free detection. *Biosens. Bioelectron.* 85: 171-177.

Singh, R., Nawale, L., Sarkar, D., Suresh, C. G. (2016). Two chitotriose-specific lectins show anti-angiogenesis, induces caspase-9-mediated apoptosis and early arrest of pancreatic tumor cell cycle. *PLoS One* 11: e0146110.

Singh, R. S., Kaur, H. P., Singh, J. (2015). Purification and characterization of a mycelial mucin specific lectin from *Aspergillus panamensis* with potent mitogenic and antibacterial activity. *Process Biochem.* 50: 2251-2258.

Srikanth, S., Chen, Z. (2016). Plant protease inhibitors in therapeutics-focus on cancer therapy. *Front. Pharmacol.* 7: 470.

Suen, Y. K., Fung, K. P., Choy, Y. M., Lee, C. Y., Chan, C. W., Kong, S. K. (2000). Concanavalin A induced apoptosis in murine macrophage PU5-1.8 cells through clustering of mitochondria and release of cytochrome c. *Apoptosis* 5: 369-377.

Sumner, J. B., Howell, S. F. (1936). Identification of hemagglutinin of jack bean with Concanavalin A. *J. Bacteriol.* 32: 227-237.

Tahirov, T. H., Lu, T. H., Liaw, Y. C., Chen, Y. L., Lin, J. Y. (1995). Crystal structure of abrin-A at 2.14 A. *J. Mol. Biol.* 250: 354-367.

Tait, S. W. G., Ichim, G., Green, D. R. (2014). Die another way--non-apoptotic mechanisms of cell death. *J. Cell Sci.* 127: 2135-2144.

Thomas, S., Fisher, K. H., Snowden, J. A., Danson, S. J., Brown, S., Zeidler, M. P. (2015). Methotrexate is a JAK/STAT pathway inhibitor. *PLoS One* 10: e0130078.

Tozawa-Ono, A., Kubota, M., Honma, C., Nakagawa, Y., Yokomichi, N., Yoshioka, N., Tsuda, C., Ohara, T., Koizumi, H., Suzuki, N. (2017). Glycan profiling using formalin-fixed, paraffin-embedded tissues: Hippeastrum hybrid lectin is a sensitive biomarker for squamous cell carcinoma of the uterine cervix. *J. Obstet. Gynaecol.* Res. 43: 1326-1334.

Trung, N. N., Tho, N. T., Thuy Dung, B. T., My Nhung, H. T., Thang, N. D. (2016). Effects of ricin extracted from seeds of the castor bean (*Ricinus communis*) on cytotoxicity and tumorigenesis of melanoma cells. Biomed. Res. Ther. 3: 633-644.

Tyagi, N., Rathore, S. S., Ghosh, P. C. (2013). Efficacy of liposomal monensin on the enhancement of the antitumour activity of liposomal ricin in human epidermoid carcinoma (KB) cells. *Indian J. Pharm. Sci.* 75, 16-22.

Tyagi, N., Tyagi, M., Pachauri, M., Ghosh, P. C. (2015). Potential therapeutic applications of plant toxin-ricin in cancer: challenges and advances. *Tumor Biol.* 36: 8239-8246.

Valentiner, U., Pfüller, U., Baum, C., Schumacher, U. (2002). The cytotoxic effect of mistletoe lectins I, II and III on sensitive and multidrug resistant human colon cancer cell lines in vitro. *Toxicology* 171: 187-199.

Varki, A., Kannagi, R., Toole, B., Stanley, P. (2017). Glycosylation changes in cancer. In: Varki, A., Cummings, R. D., Esko, J. D. et al. (Eds.), Essentials of Glycobiology, 3rd edn. Cold Spring Harbor Laboratory Press, New York, chapter 47.

Wade, M., Li, Y. C., M. Wahl, G. (2013). NF-κB, an active player in human cancers. *Nat. Rev. Cancer* 13: 83-96.

Wales, R., Richardson, P. T., Roberts, L. M., Lord, J. M. (1992). Recombinant ricin B chain fragments containing a single galactose binding site retain lectin activity. *Arch. Biochem. Biophys.* 294: 291-296.

Wallach, D., Kang, T. B., Kovalenko, A. (2014). Concepts of tissue injury and cell death in inflammation: a historical perspective. *Nat. Rev. Immunol.* 14: 51-59.

Wang, Y., Nangia-Makker, P., Balan, V., Hogan, V., Raz, A. (2010). Calpain activation through galectin-3 inhibition sensitizes prostate cancer cells to cisplatin treatment. *Cell Death Dis.* 1: e101.

Weidle, U. H., Tiefenthaler, G., Schiller, C., Weiss, E. H., Georges, G., Brinkmann, U. (2014). Prospects of bacterial and plant protein-based immunotoxins for treatment of cancer. *Cancer Gen. Proteom.* 11: 25-38.

World Health Organization (2018). Cancer statistics reports. http://www.who.int/cancer/en/ (accessed 30 March 2018).

Wu, L., Liu, T., Xiao, Y., Li, X., Zhu, Y., Zhao, Y., Bao, J., Wu, C. (2016). *Polygonatum odoratum* lectin induces apoptosis and autophagy by regulation of microRNA-1290 and microRNA-15a-3p in human lung adenocarcinoma A549 cells. *Int. J. Biol. Macromol.* 85: 217-226.

Yan, Q., Zhu, L., Kumar, N., Jiang, Z., Huang, L. (2010). Characterisation of a novel monomeric lectin (AML) from *Astragalus membranaceus* with anti-proliferative activity. *Food Chem.* 122: 589-595.

Yang, Y., Xu, H. L., Zhang, Z. T., Liu, J. J., Li, W. W., Ming, H., Bao, J. K. (2011). Characterization, molecular cloning, and in silico analysis of a novel mannose-binding lectin from *Polygonatum odoratum* (Mill.) with anti-HSV-II and apoptosis-inducing activities. *Phytomedicine* 18: 748-755.

Yau, T., Dan, X., Ng, C. C. W., Ng, T. B. (2015). Lectins with potential for anti-cancer therapy. *Molecules* 20: 3791-810.

Ye, W., Nanga, R. P., Kang, C. B., Song, J. H., Song, S. K., Yoon, H. S. (2006). Molecular characterization of the recombinant A-chain of a type II ribosome-inactivating protein (RIP) from *Viscum album* coloratum and structural basis on its ribosome-inactivating activity and the sugar-binding properties of the B-chain. *J. Biochem. Mol. Biol.* 39: 560-570.

Yue, X., Zhao, Y., Xu, Y., Zheng, M., Feng, Z., Hu, W. (2017). Mutant p53 in cancer: accumulation, gain-of-function, and therapy. *J. Mol. Biol.* 429: 1595-1606.

Zhang, Z., Peng, H., Li, C., Liu, J., Zhou, T.-T., Yan, Y., Li, Y., Bao, J. (2010). *Polygonatum cyrtonema* lectin induces murine fibrosarcoma L929 cell apoptosis via a caspase-dependent pathway as compared to *Ophiopogon japonicus* lectin. *Phytomedicine* 18: 25-31.

Zuo, Z., Fan, H., Wang, X., Zhou, W., Li, L. (2012). Purification and characterization of a novel plant lectin from Pinellia ternata with antineoplastic activity. *Springerplus* 1: 13.

Zuraidah, M. A., Mimi Sakinah, A. M., Wan Azizi, W. S. (2014). Effect of lectin from *Artocarpus heterophyllus* seed on cancer cell lines. *J. Life Sci. Technol.* 2: 55-59.

CONTENTS OF EARLIER VOLUMES

Horizons in Cancer Research. Volume 72

Horizons in Cancer Research. Volume 71

Horizons in Cancer Research. Volume 70

Horizons in Cancer Research. Volume 69

Horizons in Cancer Research. Volume 68

INDEX

A

B

C

D

E

F

G

H

I

K

L

M

N

O

P

S

T

U

V

W

X

Y

Z